FAMILY THERAPY FOR ADHD

FAMILY THERAPY FOR ADHD

Treating Children, Adolescents, and Adults

CRAIG A. EVERETT
SANDRA VOLGY EVERETT

THE GUILFORD PRESS
New York   London

#41278461

© 1999 The Guilford Press
A Division of Guilford Publications, Inc.
72 Spring Street, New York, NY 10012
http://www.guilford.com

Printed in the United States of America

This book is printed on acid-free paper.

Last digit is print number: 9 8 7 6 5 4 3 2 1

Library of Congress Cataloging-in-Publication Data

Everett, Craig A.
    Family therapy for ADHD : treating children,
adolescents, and adults / Craig A. Everett, Sandra Volgy
Everett
      p. cm.
    Includes bibliographical references and index.
    ISBN 1-57230-438-3
    1. Attention-deficit hyperactivity disorder.   2. Attention-
deficit disorder in adolescence.   3. Attention-deficit
disorder in adults.   4. Hyperactive children—Family
relationships.   5. Attention-deficit disordered children—
Family relationships.   6. Attention-deficit disordered
youth—Family relationships.   7. Attention-deficit
disordered adults—Family relationships.   8. Family
psychotherapy.   I. Volgy Everett, Sandra Sue.
II. Title.   III. Title: Family therapy for attention-deficit
hyperactivity disorder.
RJ506.H9E94   1999
616.85′89—dc21   99-30248
                                     CIP

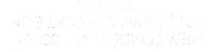

To our future generations—

Jennifer, Andrew, and Tracey Everett
Patricia Ashley Everett
Amanda Leigh Everett
Austin Gene Brunette
Bailey Everett Brunette

About the Authors

Craig A. Everett, PhD, is Director of the Arizona Institute of Family Therapy and is in private practice in Tucson, Arizona. Dr. Everett is a past president of the American Association for Marriage and Family Therapy and is Editor of *The Journal of Divorce and Remarriage*. He is the author of 14 books, most recently a trade book entitled *Healthy Divorce* and a clinical book entitled *Short-Term Family Therapy for Borderline Patients*, which he cowrote with his wife, Sandra Volgy Everett.

Sandra Volgy Everett, PhD, is Director of Clinical Education at the Arizona Institute of Family Therapy and is in private practice in Tucson, Arizona. In addition to cowriting the above books, Dr. Volgy Everett has written numerous journal articles on clinical work with children in family therapy and in divorce. She is the editor of the book *Women and Divorce/Men and Divorce*.

Acknowledgments

This book represents our accumulated experiences of over 25 years of clinical practice with children, adolescents, and their families. We want to acknowledge the ongoing learning process that we have gained from families who have had the experience of ADHD and who have allowed us to participate in their struggles and successes over the years.

We have benefited from our association with many knowledgeable and responsive colleagues. We particularly wish to acknowledge those who have played an ongoing role in our practices, with our patients, and in the preparation of this book: Howard Toff, MD, Edward Gentile, DO, Bradley Evans, MD, Michael Cohen, MD, Rebecca McReynolds, PhD, Kevin Leehey, MD, Magda Urban, PhD, and Gary Grynkewich, Esq.

We want to acknowledge and thank Marion Chacon, our office manager, for her tireless efforts in keeping our practices running smoothly while we were working on the manuscript.

Kitty Moore, Senior Editor at The Guilford Press, provided encouragement and knowledgeable feedback to help us focus and communicate our clinical experiences. Margaret Ryan, Developmental Editor, carefully reviewed and edited our entire manuscript, and we credit her with its flow and continuity.

Contents

7. Developing Therapeutic Interventions for Adolescents with ADHD and Their Families   196

8. Developing Therapeutic Interventions for Adults with ADHD and Their Families   221

References

Index

FAMILY THERAPY FOR ADHD

Family Experiences of ADHD

Attention-deficit/hyperactivity disorder (ADHD) is a complex psychiatric dysfunction that affects not only the individual who experiences the symptoms but also the individual's broader intergenerational family system. While the etiology of ADHD is based on bioneurological factors, it does not exist in a vacuum. Each family system must make accommodations to the symptomatic ADHD individual in order to maintain the family's stability and equilibrium. The necessary accommodations by the family system are often extensive and affect all family members *and* roles: parents/spouses, siblings, and grandparents. The adjustments that each family attempts to maintain, as well as the stresses and frustrations that are experienced, are present throughout the multiple subsystems and across several generations.

Given the genetic characteristics of ADHD, its diagnosis in a child becomes a "red flag" that other family members—a sibling, parent, cousin, uncle, grandfather—may also have ADHD. In families in which there are multiple ADHD members, the complexity of systemic dynamics and the need for accommodations increase exponentially.

ADHD is not contained within the boundaries of a family system. The symptomatic member experiences difficulties throughout her or his life in educational, social, and occupational endeavors. There is no cure for ADHD—but there *are* significant interventions that can normalize the ADHD individual's life experiences as well as stabilize the family system. *We believe that working with the ADHD individual in the context of her or his immediate, and even intergenerational, family system is one of the most effective clinical interventions available.*

As a psychiatric disorder, ADHD is complex and difficult to evaluate and diagnosis. However, there are effective protocols for the evaluation. We believe that conducting the evaluation—for children, adolescents, or adults—in the context of each individual's family milieu offers one of the most effective means of assessing the impact of ADHD on both the individual member (and) the overall family system. Before we explore the more technical and clinical aspects of ADHD, we will share some stories of ADHD individuals that illustrate the complexity of their struggles and the responses of their families.

Eight-year-old David slumped in his chair in the therapy session, crying. His parents had spent the last 10 minutes venting their frustration and anger at him because they believe that he is not trying in school. The school year had barely begun and David's teacher had already called his parents several times to report his failures and misdeeds. The parents' nightmare had returned. Last May the teacher and principal wanted David to repeat the second grade. His teacher had warned that he was not progressing as expected and that he was not getting along with the other students.

The parents had spent the summer investigating private schools and had decided to enroll David in a small church-sponsored elementary school was expensive and a 45-minute drive from their home. They expected improvements in David's learning level and conduct because there were only 16 students in the class and the teacher was a 20-year veteran. However, the new teacher voiced a hefty list of concerns: David was not motivated, was not completing his work, was not paying attention; would interrupt her for minor requests (such as asking for a new pencil after he had lost his own), and would interrupt the class with questions not related to the subject.

By the fourth week of school David had already been absent 10 days due to illnesses. He had been referred to the therapist (CAE) by his pediatrician, who had found no medical reasons for him to miss school. The parents believed that David was lying and that, after all they had gone through to find him a better school, he did not appreciate their efforts. They had struggled with applying many disciplinary techniques that they had read about, but to no avail—David did not improve.

David was a bright boy. When he was interviewed without his parents present, he was engaging and articulate, though somewhat sad because of his frustrations in school. He told the therapist that he loved to play on the computer and that he had taught himself how to create animated figures. He knew how to "surf" the Internet, log on to chat rooms and converse like an adult, and play at computer games designed for adults. He reported that he had been in "big" trouble during the second grade because he had installed a new screensaver and programed the school's computer to print a greeting to his teacher. Though the greeting was mildly offensive, he believed it would be a pleasant surprise for her. He said that he did not like to read books but that he was following real-life adventure reports on several websites, as well as read-

ing an encyclopedia that his father had installed on the computer—he was up to the "G's" and explained to the therapist how a gyroscope worked.

His parents had recently taken away his computer privileges as a punishment for his problems in school. They had asked the therapist, "How can he sit in front of that computer 5 hours a day and yet be unable to finish his schoolwork or pay attention in class?" In the first family session the therapist asked David to explain to his parents what he had told him about his struggles in school. At first David resisted talking about his problems and said he worried that his parents would only scold him. However, with a little prodding by the therapist, he finally tried to explain to his parents, tearfully, "I have files in my head that I can see, but sometimes I just can't keep the right information in each one."

Later in this parent–child session the therapist explained to the parents that while David was very bright and, of course, should be doing much better in school, there was a possibility that he might have ADHD. The parents looked at one another in amazement and disbelief. Both parents are high achievers. David's mother has a master's degree in education and his father operates a very successful small business with dozens of employees. David was their only child. The parents' immediate response was to deny the possibility of ADHD. By the end of the session the mother began to recognize the symptoms but became tearful about David's future. However, the father was more reflective and admitted that he has never liked to read either. In fact, he reported that he experienced difficulties early in school in both reading and writing. He wife looked at him in amazement because he had never shared this information with her, fearing that she might not think as highly of him and his success. Though he had become an excellent draftsman and owned his own company now, he had always wanted to be an architect. He had given up that dream after just 1 year of struggling in college. After further evaluation and testing, David was diagnosed with ADHD, combined type. His tests indicated that he has a Full-Scale IQ on the Wechsler Intelligence Scale for Children (WISC) of 132. Several weeks after this family session David's father called the therapist and asked to be evaluated for ADHD too.

This is a common story about the discovery of ADHD in a family. Sometimes the symptoms are recognized early, even in a toddler whose behaviors are difficult and unmanageable (hyperactive–impulsive). However, the ADHD symptoms can be subtle (inattentive type) and may not be identified until a child has struggled for several years in school, like David. Unfortunately, for many individuals who are never diagnosed, the symptoms persist throughout their school years and into their adult lives, affecting their marriages, their parenting, and their occupations.

The presence of ADHD in a family member can affect the entire family's everyday interactions and behaviors. At times its presence can profoundly affect the parents' marriage.

A month after David was diagnosed with ADHD, his father called the thera-pist and asked if he and his wife could be seen together, without David. They reported that their relationship had been in chaos since the initial diagnosis. The mother was having difficulty emotionally accepting David's ADHD, even though intellectually she had reviewed the tests and recognized the effec-tiveness of the stimulant medication on David's behavior in school. She acknowledged tearfully that she saw David as "damaged" and she blamed her husband (genetically) for this. As a child, she had lost a younger brother in a car accident, and these issues with David were causing her to relive many of those painful memories. Unfortunately, the father's early fears about reveal-ing his own school struggles were proving to be realistic, since his wife now saw him as "damaged" and had become critical of his relinquishment of a career in architecture.

An ADHD child's impulsive and hyperactive behaviors can have similar detrimental effects on parents' confidence in their management skills.

Six-year-old Billy had just entered the first grade. His parents were reviewing their difficulties with him in their initial meeting with the therapist (SVE). They described him as playful, but unlike their two older children, he had never enjoyed being cuddled. He had crawled and walked early but, after that, they could no longer contain him. He got into everything and never listened to them. At 3 years of age he was taken to an emergency room after receiving a severe gash on his arm—he had tried to climb the front of a bookcase and had pulled it over on himself, breaking a glass vase. At 4 years of age he was again taken to an emergency room after falling nearly 5 feet off a ladder that was propped against their house. The father had been working on the roof and had left the ladder in place while he went to the hardware store for supplies. They learned later that the boy had actually spent some time on the roof while the father was gone and that he fell while climbing down!

Billy had been asked to leave six different preschool programs over the previous 2 years. His teachers claimed that he was often rough and bullying with the other children. Other parents had complained about him and threat-ened to withdraw their children if Billy's conduct did not improve.

The parents acknowledged that they had fought with one another about how to handle Billy for several years. The father wanted to be tougher and more punitive with Billy "to get his attention," while the mother "kept read-ing books" and wanted to "reason with him." They indicated reported similar difficulties with their older children and they could not understand what they were doing wrong. For several years they had blamed one another for Billy's struggles. Soon their older children complained because the parents spent all their time and energy arguing about Billy.

Both parents questioned not only their functioning but even whether they should have given birth to this third child. They relived this decision many times in arguments with one another. They also acknowledged that they had stopped going out together, as well as with friends, because they continually argued about Billy. They had decided against a family vacation the prior summer because the last trip with Billy was "so horrible." They had not made love for 9 months.

Billy was diagnosed with ADHD, combined type. After several months of parent training and family therapy, Billy's behavior was improving and the parents felt more in control of their family. However, they remained in marital therapy for another 6 weeks to repair the damage to their relationship caused by the many years of their parental struggles and loss of intimacy.

The diagnosis of ADHD in a child can also cause serious sibling rivalries and confrontations in the family.

Eleven-year-old Bryan had been diagnosed with ADHD in the third grade. He was now in the fifth grade and had been medicated with a stimulant at the time of his referral. He had been quite hyperactive and impulsive, displaying reactive behaviors toward his two older siblings, teachers, and peers, and breaking objects and hitting walls. His behavior was better in school due, in part, to a smaller and well-structured classroom setting with a teacher who was effective in keeping him focused. However, his reactive behaviors still erupted periodically at home. Just before he was referred for therapy, he had become angry at his 15-year-old sister who had refused to let him enter her room. The parents were still at work. The sister felt he had been "acting wild" all afternoon and went into her room and closed the door. After 30 minutes of arguing with him to leave her alone, she locked her door and turned up her music so she could not hear him. Bryan returned with a garden pick and proceeded to smash it through her door several times. The sister was frightened and called her mother from the phone in her room. Before the mother could get home, Bryan had ripped two large holes in the sister's bedroom door. He was hiding in the back of the family's yard when the mother returned home.

In the family sessions with everyone present, the two older siblings spoke of their years of frustration and anger not only toward Bryan but toward their parents. They felt Bryan was "screwed up," and they could not understand why he received so much attention from their parents and why their parents could never control him. After the recent incident, the sister talked of wanting to live with a friend. She said that she no longer respected her parents because they never spent time with her and they could not control Bryan. She also said that when she left home, she never wanted to see Bryan again and that she would not be sad if he died.

The ADHD symptoms can intrude dramatically into a family's experience, affecting not only the child but all members of the family, as well as intergenerational relationships.

Fourteen-year-old Susan had just completed her first semester as a freshman in high school. In middle school she had received grades of C's and a few B's. Her older brother, who was more interested in sports in high school, received mostly B's. Her younger sister, who was in the sixth grade, received all A's. Susan's parents, particularly her mother, had begun to put more pressure on her to improve her grades as she began her first year of high school. However, after her first semester as a freshman, she received two F's, two D's, and three C's. Her parents were concerned and frustrated; the teachers were telling them that Susan was not reading up to grade level, she was not completing or turning in her homework, and she never seemed to be able to complete examinations.

Susan's maternal grandparents lived nearby and had a close relationship with her. However, they had told her that the money they had saved for her to go to college would be given to her sister, since she was doing so poorly. They said that her sister was the "only one in the family who cared about grades." Susan had also overheard several arguments between her mother and grandmother about her grades and had seen her mother crying afterward.

Susan's parents reported to the therapist (SVE) that they had never pushed any of their children as much as they had tried to push Susan the past year. In fact, they both reflected that they had vowed not to push their children because they had been pushed so much by their own parents. Susan's mother was particularly distraught because her mother was now accusing her of being a "bad parent" as a result of her granddaughter's failures in school. The grandparents had told her that because she had not pushed Susan, she "would never amount to anything"—and they certainly hoped she did not let the same thing happen to Mary, the youngest child. The mother was avoiding telephone calls and visits with her mother, and her husband had become angry over his in-laws' intrusions. They acknowledged that this conflict with the grandparents over Susan's grades had created the most stress between the two of them that they had ever experienced in their marriage. The husband said that he had become so angry at the grandparents and his wife, for not keeping them out of their family's life, that he had begun thinking of divorce.

The presence of ADHD in adults creates complicated layers of family dynamics and interactions, as well as associated comorbid symptoms, which can be difficult and challenging for the clinician.

In just 6 months in his practice one of the authors (CAE) had identified three adult males—ages 32 to 45—who had each been referred for therapy by their wives. These men displayed symptoms that included anger, aggression (occasional violence toward persons and property by two of the men), irritability, negativity, reactivity, moodiness, and ongoing conflict in their marriages and with their children. All three of the wives reported that their husbands displayed frequent periods of emotional unavailability toward them and their children, as well as erratic and impatient parenting behaviors.

Two of these men had been previously diagnosed with a bipolar disorder. The diagnoses had been made at 15 and 28 years of age. All of the men had been in therapy, off and on, since their diagnosis and had continued to consult with psychiatrists to monitor their medications, which included lithium, and later Depakote, as well as a variety of antidepressants. One had stayed with the original diagnosing psychiatrist while the others had changed psychiatrists, often at the urging of their spouses or friends, to seek more effective treatment. None of these men, and only one of the wives, had ever heard of ADHD. The wife who recognized the disorder reported having read some literature about it several years ago because her son's sixth grade teacher had mentioned that he might have it, but there had been no follow-up.

Two of the men were seen initially in an individual session for evaluation. Each expressed regret over his anger and occasional violence in his family and also stated that, despite a full array of pharmacological interventions and some therapy, the problem behaviors had never improved. When they were interviewed in the next session with their wives, it was learned that during the previous years of treatment and medication reviews, only twice was one of the wives interviewed by a psychiatrist. All three wives stated that they had often called their husband's psychiatrists or therapists, particularly following dramatic and unpleasant confrontations and erratic behaviors, and felt that their requests, and even pleas, for help had been rebuffed or ignored.

The joint interviews with the wives revealed a number of clinical signals—red flags—regarding the accuracy of the bipolar diagnoses and the potential for underlying (implicit) adult ADHD. After listening to the wives' reports of frustration, anger, and helpless feelings, the therapist began to evaluate the broader picture of both the husbands' early social and educational histories and their marital and family experiences.

The histories of all three men were quite similar: poor school performances (one never competed high school, one later completed his GED); frequent fights beginning as early as the fifth grade and continuing into high school (one had several assault charges as an adult, two reported slapping their wives, one reported hitting his children); drug use (two had serious problems with alcohol beginning in high school, one had serious periods of alcohol abuse as an adult) poor work histories (two of the men); and an inordinate number of traffic violations and accidents. All reported poor impulse control, which created problems in their communication and spending habits.

The wives confirmed even broader patterns of impulsivity, impatience, reactivity, moodiness, failure to start or complete projects, failure to remember conversations, failure to follow through with instructions, preoccupation with television and channel surfing, and a disinterest in playing with, or reading to, their children. While the wives reported manic-like patterns in some of these symptoms, only one identified significant periods of moodiness and depression. The information obtained in these marital interviews suggested that all three of these men had been misdiagnosed with bipolar disorders. It was also clear that subsequent clinicians and psychiatrists simply continued to accept this diagnosis without considering its accuracy or the compelling differential symptoms. This error was further exacerbated by subsequent clinicians' failure to interview the spouses and to gather data regarding the bigger picture of the individual's family milieu.

Since two of the men stated at the onset of their interviews that they had been diagnosed with bipolar disorder, the therapist was not expecting underlying ADHD issues. The early red flag was the men's indication that they had "done everything possible," "taken every pill" they had been given, "tried to control" themselves better at home, and nothing had improved. In fact, two of the men indicated clearly that they had never experienced beneficial effects from the variety of medications they had taken over the years.

The warning signals of ADHD may have been missed if the marital interviews had not further explored the behavioral patterns and symptomatology. As part of the ensuing evaluation, two telephone interviews—the first with one of the men's father, his only living parent; and the second with the other man's parents and a brother—were conducted. These family-of-origin consultations, as we will discuss in later chapters, provided important childhood observations and histories that only parents could make available. The information gained from these interviews corroborated the ADHD diagnoses. The interaction with extended family members also revealed that one of the men's fathers and potentially two siblings had displayed ADHD symptoms. It was also learned in subsequent interviews that two of the three families had children with ADHD symptoms.

Following the preliminary ADHD diagnoses, the three men were seen by two psychiatric colleagues regarding the diagnostic issues and possible changes in their medications. All three men were placed on stimulant medications and the one who had displayed some depression was continued on a previously prescribed antidepressant. All three wives, within days, reported dramatic changes in their husbands. Most notably, they reported that their husbands' unrelenting intensity had subsided. One wife called the therapist within 3 days to say that she was amazed that her husband was able to sit still for more than 5 minutes and actually carry on a conversation with her. Another wife called, tearfully reporting that she had come home from work the previous day to find her husband playing quietly on the floor with their 7-year-old daughter. She said this was the first time she had ever seen him do that.

They participated in family therapy sessions that included their children. Those children suspected of also having ADHD were evaluated and a treatment plan was developed for them. Subsequent marital sessions were helpful in repairing the damage of distrust, hurt, and lost intimacy. The family sessions were instrumental in helping the children understand their fathers' disorders and their previous behaviors, as well as a beginning step toward repairing parent–child trust.

As we have illustrated in these case overviews, we believe it is essential that both the evaluation and the resulting treatment plan occur in the context of the ADHD individual's family milieu. To accomplish this, the therapist must learn to listen to the struggles of *all* the family members, respecting their observations as well as their own unique resources for change. We have been in clinical practice, for nearly 25 years and have learned that all families, no matter how dysfunctional they may appear, have inherent resources that can be mobilized to affect lasting change. These resources may have been camouflaged or buried for years under conflict, but the skilled family therapist learns to sort through these subterfuges to reveal the issues and create healthier interactional experiences.

As a result of our experience in working with families, we have always focused on the child's symptomatology as a window into the clinical dynamics of the entire family. Even before the development of the ADHD diagnosis, we were working with families to contain and manage the hyperactive behaviors of a single child and the resulting impact on siblings and the marital relationship. We have learned much from the ADHD families with whom we have worked, and, in our experience have found *family therapy to be the most effective treatment of choice*. In the following chapters we describe our methods of evaluating and treating ADHD individuals—children, adolescents, and adults—in the contexts of their family systems.

1

Diagnosing ADHD
in Clinical Practice

ADHD affects people of all ages, of both genders, and from a diversity of cultural and racial backgrounds. When ADHD patients come into the clinician's office, they will often present a variety of recognizable ADHD symptoms. These symptoms typically appear in what we refer to as "clusters." For the clinician who has limited experience working with ADHD and its multiple comorbid clinical symptoms, it is important to recognize these clusters of ADHD symptoms as their appear across the developmental range of children, adolescents, and adults. Some ADHD patients may present symptoms that cannot be identified immediately by the therapist, given the patient's age and relative developmental level. These same patients may also have comorbid psychiatric symptoms that camouflage or exacerbate the underlying ADHD symptoms. Often these additional psychiatric symptoms, such as depression or oppositional behaviors, will overshadow the often more subtle ADHD symptoms. Therapists who work with couples and families may also be surprised to detect ADHD symptoms in parents and other family members across several generations. As we have indicated, it is important for the clinician to understand and identify the ADHD disorder in the context of the individual's history and presenting symptomatology and from the perspective of his or her broader family and social interactional milieu.

The presence of the ADHD disorder will also shape the interactional patterns and roles among family members for several generations. We will discuss how ADHD symptoms create patterns of low self-esteem and poor social and academic skills in a child, which, in turn, evoke frustrated parental responses that may take the form of scapegoating the ADHD child. These parental failures may then lead to serious marital problems. The ADHD symptoms may also circum-

11

scribe the child's developmental experiences across the life cycle, influencing his or her sense of self-esteem and identity, social skills and dating, mate selection, and future parenting role. Whether one works primarily with children, adolescents, or adults, it is important for the clinician to be cognizant of the subtleties of the ADHD diagnostic criteria as well as the ongoing literature and research regarding the disorder's neurobiological etiology and behavioral manifestations that inform both assessment and treatment. Since the ADHD field is relatively new and still evolving, the literature often contains contradictory and even controversial hypotheses and theoretical formulations.

In this chapter we will:

1. Review the history of the ADHD diagnosis.
2. Identify the present DSM-IV diagnostic criteria for ADHD and review the ongoing critique of these criteria.
3. Discuss what causes ADHD (etiology) and how it can be transmitted intergenerationally among family members.
4. Review the occurrence of ADHD in various populations (epidemiology).
5. Identify other disorders that can occur with ADHD (comorbidity).
6. Discuss the diagnosis and symptoms of ADHD in adults, along with possible comorbid disorders.

A BRIEF HISTORY OF ADHD

The cluster of symptoms that define our present understanding of ADHD was first recognized by medical and psychiatric practitioners in the late 19th century. Their early observations primarily concerned behaviors in individuals who had experienced neurological damage either through trauma or central nervous system infections. The emergence and identification of these symptom clusters in this country followed an encephalitis epidemic in the early 1900s. These postrecovery encephalitic patients, as well as other posttrauma patients, displayed behaviors that typically included hyperactivity, impulsivity, and distractibility. These primary symptoms became the base of the definition of the new disorder, which was originally termed brain damage. However, by 1940 A. A. Strauss had suggested that this cluster of behaviors might also exist independently of specific neurological injury or infectious disease. He hypothesized that these symptoms represented evidence of more specific brain damage. These and other observations led to the renaming of this syndrome as *minimal brain damage*. Some years later its name was changed again to *minimal brain dysfunction* (MBD) (Interagency Committee in Learning Disabilities, 1987; Routh, 1983).

Through the 1950s MBD was used primarily to designate hyperactive behaviors in the absence of concurrent neurological trauma. Other terms in use during this period were *hyperkinesis* and the *hyperactive child syndrome* (Wender, 1995). After 1960 the clinical use of the term was broadened to include learning disabilities, general neurological dysfunctions, and other behavioral symptoms. With the appearance of the second edition of the *Diagnostic and Statistical Manual of Mental Disorders* (DSM-II; American Psychiatric Association, 1968), learning disabilities were separated into an additional category and the MBD behavioral symptoms comprised primarily those associated with hyperactivity.

The identification of these symptoms has evolved from early efforts to describe broad clinical phenomena to the present consensus concerning six specific symptomatic behaviors: *hyperactivity, restlessness, impulsivity, aggression, distractibility,* and *short attention span*. With the appearance of the DSM-III (American Psychiatric Association, 1980), these six symptoms were further refined into the definition of ADHD. Here the six symptoms were categorized according to three specific behavioral patterns: *hyperactivity, impulsivity,* and *inattention*. In the DSM-III the incidence of ADHD was estimated at approximately 3% of the childhood population. It was also estimated at that time that ADHD appeared predominantly in males (with an estimated predominance between 6:1 and 9:1) and that approximately one-third of these ADHD children would continue to display symptoms in their adult years.

The most dramatic step in expanding the clinical understanding and definition of ADHD occurred some years later with the recognition *that ADHD can occur in children and adults in which the classic symptoms of hyperactivity are either less prominent or nonexistent while the symptoms of inattentiveness continue to be present*. For nearly a century the primary defining symptom of our current ADHD diagnosis was hyperactivity. With the publication of the DSM-III in 1980 (American Psychiatric Association), a new generation of children could now be diagnosed without the previously necessary presence of hyperactive behaviors.

These ADHD children who do not display hyperactivity are often described by their parents or teachers as "spacey or daydreaming" but not a behavior problem. To the clinician, these children may appear to be similar to anxiety disordered children, who are dependent, socially passive, and immature. However, as we will discuss later, the clinical discrimination of these nonhyperactive ADHD children remains a continuing challenge for therapists and educators alike.

Further research and definition of this new category of "ADHD without hyperactivity" did not evolve for some years. The primary symptoms of inattentiveness are often subtle and can be masked by a child's innate intelligence and other cognitive resources. A study from Israel (Bar-Josef et al., 1995) reported that children with ADHD *inattentive type* often "escape accurate diagnosis" because their symptoms are not conspicuous and their natural intelligence may compensate for learning problems. It has been our observation, which is supported by some preliminary research, that many of these children are never diagnosed until they enter middle school where larger classes, multiple teachers, and more complex educational assignments can create overwhelming distractions and stressors. The more recent DSM-IV (American Psychiatric Association, 1994) classification and definition of ADHD provides the practitioner with even more specificity to aid in making the diagnosis of these children: *attention-deficit/hyperactivity disorder, predominantly inattentive type (314.00).*

Before we discuss the specific DSM-IV ADHD diagnostic criteria, it may be helpful for the reader to understand that Barkley (1990a, 1990b), in research that predated the diagnostic additions in the DSM-IV, had already compared groups of ADHD children with and without hyperactivity and suggested that these two types might be distinct disorders rather than just subtypes of a single disorder. He reported that the ADHD children *with hyperactivity* displayed more externalizing and internalizing symptoms and were more distracted during testing. This group of hyperactive children also reported a higher frequency of substance abuse and aggression by other family members than did the groups of ADHD children without hyperactivity, ADHD children with learning disabilities, and children in the control group. The ADHD children *without hyperactivity* displayed more patterns of daydreaming, lethargy, impaired perceptual–motor speed, and anxiety disorders. Morgan and associates (1996) reported that ADHD children with the combined subtype, which involves the presence of both the hyperactive–impulsive symptoms and the inattentive symptoms, displayed more externalizing comorbid diagnoses, as well as more delinquent and aggressive behaviors, than children in the other subtypes. These studies have aided the ongoing discussions and debates in the field regarding the differentiation of the subtypes and the question as to whether these are genuine subtypes or discrete disorders.

The addition of the new diagnostic categories and criteria in the DSM-IV has engendered criticism and created controversy in the field. Barkley (1997), who is widely recognized as being at the forefront of ADHD research and theory, has suggested that the theoretical model underlying the DSM-IV criteria for ADHD may be inadequate and that there is a need for the field to develop a new model. He contends that the present categories defining the subtypes of ADHD are flawed in that they assume similar deficits in attention to be present in each subtype, with the differentiation based on the presence of hyperactive–impulsive symptoms. He hypothesizes that the hyperactive–impulsive type may be simply a "developmental precursor" to the combined type and that *the hyperactive–impulsive and combined types may be specifically distinct disorders from the inattentive type.* The former types appear to have an earlier onset, in preschool years, while the inattentive type only becomes apparent some years later. He believes that the hyperactive–impulsive types reflect problems specifically with disinhibition and executive functions of self-regulation *but not inattention,* whereas the symptoms associated with inattentive types (daydreaming, lethargy, hypoactivity, passivity, "spacing out," and deficits in speed of processing information) are characteristically different.

THE DSM-IV DIAGNOSIS

Since practitioners continue to express confusion about and consequent difficulty in using the DSM-IV diagnostic criteria for ADHD, we will now review the categories and definitions for our reader. The DSM-IV (American Psychiatric Association, 1994, p. 80) defines the three basic subtypes of ADHD in the following manner:

314.01 Attention-deficit/hyperactivity disorder, combined type. This diagnosis describes individuals whose symptoms include aspects of all three behaviors: inattentiveness, hyperactivity, and impulsivity. This subtype may be used if six or more symptoms occur representing both inattention and hyperactivity/impulsivity for 6 months.

314.00 Attention-deficit/hyperactivity disorder, predominantly inattentive type. This diagnosis describes individuals whose symptoms are primarily those of inattention and distractibility, rather than impulsivity or hyperactivity. This subtype may be used if six or more symptoms of inattention have persisted over six months, but fewer than 6 symptoms of hyperactivity–impulsivity are present.

314.01 Attention-deficit/hyperactivity disorder, predominantly hyperactive–impulsive type. This diagnostic group includes those individuals whose symptoms are primarily those of hyperactivity and impulsivity rather than inattention. This subtype may be used if six or more symptoms of hyperactivity or impulsivity have been present for 6 months, but fewer than six symptoms of inattention are present.

While not a subtype, the following category is also included in DSM-IV (American Psychiatric Association, 1994, p. 85):

> 314.9 Attention-deficit/hyperactivity disorder, not otherwise specified. This category describes individuals who display ADHD symptoms as a result of closed-head traumas, illnesses such as encephalitis, or damage from environmental toxins such as lead. It may also be used to describe older adults (+60) who cannot recall their early history, or individuals who do not meet the complete criteria above.

The DSM-IV has outlined the following 18 criteria (nine represent inattentive behaviors and nine represent hyperactivity/impulsivity behaviors) to support the diagnosis of ADHD. The diagnosis requires the presence of a minimum of *six* of the following symptoms for at least a period of *6 months*. Additional requirements specify that the symptoms must be more disruptive than similar behavioral patterns normally found in the same-age population and they must be serious enough to impair the child's functioning in more than one setting, for example, home and school. In addition, the clinician is required to establish that some of these symptoms must have existed since *before the age of 7*. This latter criterion has become quite controversial and will be discussed later. The criteria are as follows:

Inattention
  (a) often fails to give close attention to details or makes careless mistakes in schoolwork, work, or other activities
  (b) often has difficulty sustaining attention in tasks or play activities
  (c) often does not seem to listen when spoken to directly
  (d) often does not follow through on instructions and fails to finish schoolwork, chores, or duties in the workplace (not due to oppositional behavior or failure to understand instructions)
  (e) often has difficulty organizing tasks and activities
  (f) often avoids, dislikes, or is reluctant to engage in tasks that require sustained mental effort (such as schoolwork or homework)
  (g) often loses things necessary for tasks or activities (e.g., toys, school assignments, pencils, books, or tools)
  (h) is often easily distracted by extraneous stimuli
  (i) is often forgetful in daily activities

Hyperactivity
(a) often fidgets with hands or feet or squirms in seat
(b) often leaves seat in classroom or in other situations in which remaining seated is expected
(c) often runs about or climbs excessively in situations in which it is inappropriate (in adolescents or adults, may be limited to subjective feelings of restlessness)
(d) often has difficulty playing or engaging in leisure activities quietly
(e) is often "on the go" or often acts as if "driven by a motor"
(f) often talks excessively

Impulsivity
(g) often blurts out answers before questions have been completed
(h) often has difficulty awaiting turn
(i) often interrupts or intrudes on others (e.g., butts into conversations or games) (American Psychiatric Association, 1994, pp. 83–84)

These criteria differentiate fairly clearly between the predominantly inattentive and the hyperactive–impulsive subtypes. In many cases the differentiation among these subtypes will be easy to make, particularly regarding hyperactive children. However, the therapist will need to learn to look carefully for the more subtle patterns of inattention that may exist in very bright children who do not display the symptoms of hyperactivity. Many of these children may never be diagnosed with ADHD. The combined subtype is designed to include the child who displays a broader range of ADHD symptoms that span all three areas: inattention, hyperactivity, and impulsivity. This subtype tends to be used more frequently with younger children simply because it can be more difficult to differentiate the various symptoms in this age group. It may also be used with ADHD adults who display milder forms of both hyperactivity and inattention.

Unfortunately, differentiating among these diagnostic criteria for children, adolescents, and adults can be extremely difficult. For the therapist who works primarily with children, the list of 18 criteria may be frustratingly familiar because it describes many typical childhood behaviors. For the therapist who works predominantly with adolescents or adults, the criteria will need to be skillfully interpreted and translated regarding the behavioral variations for older adolescents, young adults, and older adults. In our clinical chapters we include discussion designed to assist clinicians in understanding and diagnosing ADHD among differing age populations.

The criterion requiring the clinician to establish that significant ADHD symptoms were present and causing an "impairment" prior to the age of 7, which was carried over from the DSM-III to the DSM-IV, is controversial. To meet this diagnostic requirement for children and adolescents, clinicians must rely heavily upon reflections and reports provided by parents. Of course, this requirement makes the diagnosis of ADHD in adults especially difficult, since parental reports are often unavailable or unreliable. The other controversial diagnostic issue concerns the relative timing of the appearance of ADHD symptoms as compared to the determination of when "impairment" may have actually occurred. Studies have now shown that the actual age of onset of ADHD symptoms can be quite variable.

In a study of 45 ADHD male and female children, all 11 years old, McGee and associates (1992) reported that the comparative ages of onset were equally distributed: one-third of the cohort by 3 years of age, another one-third by 5 to 6 years of age (also defined as the first year of school), and one-third by 6 to 7 years of age (defined as the end of the second year of school). An extensive study by Applegate and colleagues (1997) found that parents of ADHD children and adolescents tended to report the presence of ADHD symptoms 2½ years prior to the actual onset of impairment. This finding seemed to suggest that ADHD impairments per se are identified more readily by parents *after* a child has become involved in school experiences, which create and demonstrate struggles and frustrations. For many ADHD children, particularly the inattentive type, the educational demands that eventually produce impairments may not occur until the child has reached later grade levels.

These and other researchers in the field have questioned the validity of the DSM-IV's diagnostic criteria and concluded that the focus on the "age of onset of impairment" rather than the age of onset of symptoms "may have been a mistake" (Applegate et al., 1997, p. 1220). Applegate and his associates (1997) also observed that most of the clinicians diagnosing ADHD either did not apply or simply ignored this age-of-onset criterion, while others purposefully focused on the age of onset of the symptoms. Barkley and Biederman (1997) presented an even stronger critique. While they acknowledge support for viewing ADHD symptoms as arising during childhood, they argue that there is no solid support for the selection of age 7 as defining either onset of symptoms or onset of impairments: "Several reasons favor dispensing with a precise AOC [age-of-onset criterion, either for symptom onset or for onset of impairment, not the least of which is that it is scientifically indefensible, poses unwarranted practical problems for the study of older adolescents and adults, and may be arbitrarily discriminatory" (p. 1204). Our diagnostic experiences confirm the dilemma created by this criterion, and we tend to follow the latter choice of identifying the age of onset of symptoms.

As a supplement to the DSM-IV, the Diagnostic and Statistical

Manual for Primary Care, Child and Adolescent Version (DSM-PC; American Academy of Pediatrics, 1996) has been developed to identify subclinical populations of children and adolescents whose symptoms do not meet the DSM-IV criteria for diagnosing formal disorders. This is a useful guide for the practitioner because it recognizes both the interactive influences of a child or adolescent with his or her environment and "developmental variations." The manual identifies five behaviors related to ADHD: (1) hyperactive/impulsivity, (2) inattention, (3) negative emotions, (4) aggression/opposition, and (5) secretive antisocial. While this resource has neither been widely used nor subjected to empirical studies, it does assist the therapist in recognizing the broader range of ADHD symptoms.

It is important for the clinician who is just beginning to work in the ADHD field to understand both the diagnostic dilemmas and the varying points of view regarding the implementation of the criteria. The fact that there is a continuing debate concerning these issues reflects the ongoing evolution of both diagnostic and treatment strategies in a relatively new field. We will discuss some of these issues further in the following chapters.

RESEARCH AND THEORIES ON ADHD

Many therapists in clinical practice struggle with finding the time to keep abreast of new research. Yet new data can have profound effects on one's clinical practice. Keeping informed about the research and theory regarding ADHD is particularly critical because the field continues to evolve and the etiology of the disorder is clearly rooted in biochemical and medical phenomena. An awareness of the ongoing flow of substantive research will continue to inform and help the therapist refine his or her diagnostic and treatment skills. In addition, while the therapist does not need to become an "expert" in neurobiological phenomena, he or she should be conversant with the findings and studies, which will help therapists better inform ADHD patients and their families about this disorder. Specific benefits of understanding the research and theory on ADHD for clinical practice include:

- Understanding the biochemical processes underlying the ADHD cluster of symptoms.
- Recognizing how different medications affect symptoms.
- Learning to differentiate the intertwined psychological and biological symptoms.
- Understanding how the disorder can be transmitted over several generations.

- Recognizing the disorder's epidemiology.
- Recognizing other symptoms and disorders that appear with ADHD (comorbidity).
- Becoming more effective in making differential diagnoses.
- Learning to differentiate symptom clusters that appear in ADHD children, adolescents, and adults.

Since the literature in these areas is extensive, we will give readers a guided tour of the data that we believe is the most relevant for clinical practice and, wherever possible, we will identify further resources where one can pursue certain studies or issues more thoroughly.

In the following sections we will discuss:

- The present theories of what causes ADHD.
- How the disorder is transmitted over generations and appears in other family members.
- Disinhibition and dysregulation.
- MRI, SPECT, and PET studies.
- Epidemiology of the disorder.
- Comorbidity of ADHD with other disorders such as depression, conduct and oppositional disorder, anxiety, substance abuse, and learning difficulties.

ETIOLOGY

A specific etiology for ADHD remains undefined, though dramatic progress has been made in the past decade through neurobiological research. Most studies concur that there is a clear genetic transmission factor in most cases of ADHD. Nongenetic cases involve traumatic brain injuries or serious illness that might damage or alter brain chemistry. The focus of much of the neurobiological research is on genetic and intergenerational familial transmission (Biederman et al., 1986, 1989, 1990, 1992; Cantwell, 1972; Faraone et al., 1991; Gittelman et al., 1985; Morrison & Stewart, 1971, 1973; Weiss et al., 1985).

Frick and associates (1991) reported that in a study of the biological relatives of ADHD boys ages 7 to 12, the parents and relatives displayed a significant history of childhood ADHD. Biederman and associates (1986) reported that ADHD appeared in as large a proportion as 31.5% of first-degree relatives of ADHD male children and adolescents as compared to its occurrence in only 5.7% of the relatives of a control group. Similarly, Robin and associates (1995) reviewed ADHD information from 85 families involving a total of 355 family members.

They reported that 42% had been diagnosed with ADHD (24 fathers, 22 mothers, 80 sons, 25 daughters), while another 19% were suspected of having ADHD. The combined figure was a dramatic 61% of family members who had either been diagnosed with or suspected of having ADHD.

These findings, highly suggestive of genetic involvement, have been supported by other studies, including those of twins (Gilles et al., 1992; Goodman & Stevenson, 1989) and of adopted children (Barkley, 1990a). While as yet no specific contributing gene has been identified, one study identified the dopamine D-2 receptor as a modifying factor in 46% of a group of ADHD individuals (Comings et al., 1991).

The implication of these findings for clinicians is clear: numerous biological relatives across an intergenerational span may also have ADHD symptoms. This is an important reality clinically for two reasons. First, the initial diagnosis of an ADHD child or adult should alert clinicians to the need for screening other family members. Second, clinical and/or educational interventions must recognize and include these other members. Treatment cannot be limited solely to the diagnosed child or adult, as has been mistakenly suggested in much of the literature.

Much of the recent research regarding the etiology of ADHD has focused on the neurobiological functions of *disinhibition* and *dysregulation*. The structures that mediate these functions are located in the frontal cortex. These studies have suggested that hyperactivity is the direct result of "cortical inhibition" (Barkley et al., 1992; Chelune et al., 1986; Douglas, 1984; Quinn, 1997). Early EEG studies reported abnormal brain waves in the frontal lobe of ADHD children (Lubar et al., 1985). Other studies used the resources of electronic imaging techniques, including SPECT (single photon emission computed tomography) and PET (positron emission tomography). In the PET studies (Cantwell, 1994; Zametkin et al., 1993; Zametkin et al., 1990), ADHD adults who had an ADHD child displayed lower cerebral glucose metabolism in the promotor cortex and the superior prefrontal cortex, the areas of the brain that control attention and motor activity. However, a strong association was not found for ADHD adolescent males. ADHD adolescent females displayed a lower glucose metabolism than either a normal male/female control group or ADHD males. Similar MRI (magnetic resonance imaging) studies have identified in ADHD children both differences in the frontal lobe and in the size and morphology of the corpus callosum (Hynd et al., 1990). Other MRI studies have also located anatomic asymmetries in ADHD boys (Castellanos et al., 1996).

Dopamine is considered to be a central biochemical factor in ADHD etiology. The presence and influence of dopamine in the motor cortex and other prefrontal areas of the brain are seen as critical to the functioning of the frontal lobe. Impairment in this lobe inhibits blood flow and metabolism which, in turn, diminishes control from the lower brain structures, thereby potentially producing the ADHD symptoms (Quinn, 1997; Zametkin & Rapoport, 1987).

A variety of hypotheses or "myths" have been presented over the years to explain the causes of ADHD. It has been proposed, for example, that excessive sugar intake or food additives, lead toxins, or deficiencies in nutrition and vitamins could be causative factors. However, the research has not supported any of these suggested influences (Arnold & Jensen, 1995; Barkley, 1990a; Behar et al., 1984; Cantwell, 1996).

While it has been assumed in some of the literature (and we concur) that family dynamics and psychosocial factors are not directly involved in the specific etiology of ADHD (Cantwell, 1996), this does not mean that family dynamics do not play a crucial role in an ADHD individual's emotional and behavioral responses to the disorder. For example, the endless strain of caring for an ADHD child can contribute to symptoms such as anxiety, depression, or emotional withdrawal in parents or siblings. Later in this book we will identify how the cluster of behaviors associated with ADHD in both children and adults, whether or not they have been diagnosed as ADHD, can evoke a circular series of responses from the individual's nuclear and intergenerational family, as well as from peers and caregivers in the community.

EPIDEMIOLOGY

Overall estimates of the occurrence of ADHD in the population of school-age children range from 3% to 5% by some sources (American Psychiatric Association, 1994; Cantwell, 1996) and 6% to 9% by others (Wilens et al., 1995b). A recent study utilizing the DSM-IV criteria among a general school-age population in Tennessee identified the following incidence of ADHD: inattentive, 4.7%; hyperactive, 3.4%; and combined, 4.4% (Wolraich et al., 1996). A similar German study reported a somewhat higher incidence: inattentive, 9.0%; hyperactive, 3.9%; and combined, 4.8% (Baumgaertel et al., 1995).

The early estimates of gender differences in ADHD populations were rather dramatic, suggesting a ratio potentially as high as 9:1, males to females. More recent epidemiological samples have suggested a less dramatic ratio of 4:1. There are, of course, selective issues here, in that males more commonly display the hyperactive and impulsive symptoms related to behavioral disturbances and conduct disorders. Thus, these males tend to be referred more frequently for clinical services (Cantwell, 1994, 1996; Wolraich et al., 1996).

Quinn (1997) has pointed out that as clinicians have become more familiar with the newer DSM-IV category of inattention, girls have been diagnosed with ADHD in increasing numbers. She suggested that the male : female ratio may be as low as 3:1 or even 2:1. A recent study of an ADHD population using the DSM-IV criteria found the following proportions of girls in each category: inattentive, 27%; hyperactive, 20%; and combined, 12% (McBurnett, 1995).

Overall, studies of ADHD girls have indicated that they (1) do not manifest the typical symptoms of hyperactivity and impulsivity (Berry et al., 1985); (2) display more cognitive impairments, particularly in language functioning (Berry et al., 1985); (3) tend to internalize and therefore display more symptoms of anxiety and depression (Brown et al., 1989); (4) have more learning problems, are later referrals, and experience more peer rejection (O'Brien et al., 1994; Phillips et al., 1993); and (5) report an exacerbation of mood swings with the onset of puberty and their menstrual cycle (Hussey, 1990). We have summarized these differential patterns in Table 1.1.

COMORBIDITY

One of the most important developments in both clinical studies and diagnostic procedures, a development that will greatly aid the therapist's role in evaluation and differential diagnosis, has been the recognition that most individuals with ADHD, both children and adults, also display other serious diagnosable psychiatric disorders. In fact, in many ADHD individuals symptoms for these comorbid conditions are more clearly identifiable than their ADHD symptoms. Of course, this

TABLE 1.1. Differential Symptoms of ADHD Girls

Symptom	Research
Cognitive impairments	Berry et al. (1985)
Internalization	Brown et al. (1989)
Anxiety	Brown et al. (1989)
Depression	Brown et al. (1989)
Learning problems	O'Brien et al. (1994); Phillips et al. (1993)
Peer rejection	O'Brien et al. (1994); Phillips et al. (1993)
Delayed referrals	O'Brien et al. (1994); Phillips et al. (1993)
Exacerbated mood swings with puberty and menstruation	Hussey (1990)

complicates the evaluation process for the clinician and enhances the need for care in making differential diagnoses. In this section we will clarify the relationship of these other disorders to ADHD. We will also highlight the importance of recognizing the "red flags" of ADHD when they occur in either children or adults who have been referred primarily for other problematic behaviors, such as conduct disorders, affective disorders, or learning disabilities (LD).

Biederman and his associates (1987) conducted 1-year and 4-year follow-up studies on groups of ADHD children and control cohorts, and found that the ADHD children were "at high risk" for a variety of psychopathological impairments in the areas of cognition, interpersonal relationships, and school and family functioning. Studies have also indicated that as many as two-thirds of ADHD elementary school children referred for clinical evaluations may also display other psychiatric disorders. In addition, it has been reported that the severity of the hyperactivity component in both boys and girls can be a predictor of the incidence and range of comorbid symptoms (Gabel et al., 1996). In an early control study Munir and associates (1987) found that ADHD boys, ages 5 through 16, displayed higher rates of conduct disorders, oppositional disorders, major affective disorder, tics, enuresis, and learning difficulties than a similar control group.

Many studies have concluded that the most common comorbid disorders diagnosed in connection with ADHD in children and adolescents are conduct disorder and oppositional defiant disorder. As Munir's (1987) research reported, other typical diagnoses include anxiety and mood disorders, language and learning disorders, and Tourette's syndrome. Substance abuse and obsessive–compulsive disorders have been added (Biederman et al., 1991, 1992, 1993; Cantwell, 1996, 1994). Barkley (1990a) suggested that as many as 75% of children and adolescents diagnosed with ADHD will display symptoms of depression into adulthood. He has also indicated that 27% may abuse alcohol and 23–45% may become juvenile offenders with convictions. An outpatient study reported that one-third of children with ADHD had also been diagnosed with either conduct disorder or oppositional defiant disorder (Carlson, 1986). The most common comorbid psychiatric disorders present in ADHD children and adolescents are listed in Table 1.2.

Conduct and Oppositional Defiant Disorders

Conduct and oppositional disorders are the most common comorbid diagnoses for ADHD children and adolescents. A *conduct disorder* diagnosis requires a repetitive and persistent pattern of behavior involving

TABLE 1.2. Psychiatric Disorders Comorbid with Childhood and Adolescent ADHD

1. Conduct disorder	6. Affective disorders
2. Oppositional defiant disorder	7. Anxiety disorders
3. Depression (nonpsychotic)	8. Polydrug abuse/addiction
4. Dysthymia	9. Alcohol abuse/addiction
5. Bipolar disorders	10. Learning disabilities

the violation of rules or the rights of others through aggressive actions directed at people and/or animals (physical cruelty and fighting, destruction of property, vandalism, stealing, setting fires, a disregard for rules by ignoring parental curfews, being truant from school, or runaway behavior). Barkley (1990a) reported that between 20% and 30% of preadolescent ADHD children and between 40% and 60% of ADHD adolescents meet the diagnostic criteria for conduct disorder. In a follow-up study of ADHD children, Barkley (1990a) reported that 43% had been diagnosed with conduct disorder.

A similar study reported that the presence of ADHD significantly predicted the diagnosis of conduct disorder in boys ages 8 to 17 (Loeber et al., 1995). Soltys and associates (1992) reported that in an inpatient group of ADHD children, ages 7 to 12, those with a comorbid diagnosis of conduct disorder demonstrated greater degrees of psychopathology than other groups of ADHD children. Similarly, Walker and associates (1987) reported that subjects with both ADHD and conduct disorder displayed greater physical aggression and more severe antisocial behaviors. In a comparative study, O'Brien and associates (1992) reported that children with the joint diagnosis of ADHD and conduct disorder performed significantly more poorly in academic achievement than a similar group of conduct-disordered subjects only.

Among studies of child and adolescent delinquency, Zagar and associates (1989) studied a sample of 1,956 adjudicated subjects, males and females ages 6 to 17, and identified 9% as having ADHD with hyperactivity and 46% as having ADHD without hyperactivity. Moffitt and Silva (1988) found that in a group of 13-year-old ADHD boys, the ones who had been classified in the general category of "delinquency" displayed greater memory difficulties and greater cognitive impairment than the ADHD nondelinquent boys.

The *oppositional defiant disorder* is somewhat less severe than conduct disorder and involves problematic attitudes rather than destructive behaviors. These children and adolescents display noncompliance, hostility, and stubbornness toward parents, teachers, and others in authority. Barkley (1990a) reported that up to 65% of children with

ADHD meet the criteria for this diagnosis. The findings of a comparative clinical study, which identified groups of oppositional only, ADHD only, comorbid, and a control group of 6- to 12-year-old boys, supported the importance of recognizing the comorbidity of these diagnoses and reported that the comorbid group was more greatly impaired than the control group (Paternite et al., 1995).

An interesting 9-year follow-up study of ADHD boys predicted their later arrest records (Satterfield et al., 1994). The authors used a defiance rating measure to study drug-treated ADHD boys, multimodality-treated ADHD boys, and a normal control group of boys. The dramatic findings indicated that the ADHD boys with the highest defiance ratings had significantly higher juvenile felony offender rates. Even the ADHD boys with lower defiance ratings had higher felony rates than boys in the control group. The authors observed that the defiance component in ADHD boys is certainly a "signal" for increased risk of later antisocial behavior, and argued that this potential should be considered even in ADHD boys with lower levels of defiance.

Faraone and associates (1995), who studied ADHD children and their siblings in relation to specific family typologies, found that children from families that were classified as "antisocial" displayed greater psychopathology. The authors suggested that antisocial disorders "signal a distinct subtype of ADHD." Barkley and Anastopoulos (1992), in a comparative study of ADHD adolescents with and without the oppositional defiant characteristics, reported that the latter group displayed "greater than normal" conflicts, more anger, poorer communication, and negative interactional styles, and that their mothers reported significantly greater parental distress and hostility.

Mood Disorders

A specific relationship between the co-occurrence of ADHD and mood disorders remains unclear, though studies have reported a high incidence of affective symptoms among ADHD children (Jensen et al., 1988). Biederman and associates (1987) reported a comorbidity of depression with ADHD as high as 25%. An outpatient clinic reported that one-third of their ADHD children were diagnosed with either mood or anxiety disorders. An inpatient study of ADHD children, ages 5 to 18, reported that 68% met the criteria for mood disorders: 36% nonpsychotic depression, 8% psychotic depression, and 22% bipolar disorder (Butler et al., 1995). Angold and Costello (1993), in a review of epidemiological studies, reported an incidence of ADHD as high as 57% in studies of children and adolescents with either a major mood disorder or dysthymia.

In a study of inpatient children and adolescents, ages 5 to 18, Butler and associates (1995) reported that 66% of the ADHD subjects were diagnosed with a mood disorder (36% with nonpsychotic depression, 8% with psychotic depression, and 22% with bipolar disorder). Very few studies have investigated the presence of comorbid depression in ADHD adults. (Issues of differential diagnosis with comorbid mood disorders, particularly with bipolar disorder, will be discussed in another section.)

Anxiety Disorders

Coexisting anxiety disorders in ADHD children have been reported at rates up to 25% (Biederman et al., 1991). Higher rates of anxiety disorders were also observed by Lahey and associates (1987) in ADHD children without hyperactivity. Carlson (1986) reported that one-third of an outpatient clinic population of ADHD children, which he studied, were diagnosed with either anxiety or mood disorders.

Substance Abuse

Any clinician who has worked in this area recognizes that ADHD adolescents, a growing number of ADHD preadolescents, and ADHD adults are at risk for a variety of substance abuse problems. In our practices we have observed that up to 50% of the adolescents and adults we have worked with who began treatment based on substance abuse problems, had already been, or will be, diagnosed with ADHD. Quinn (1997), in reviewing eight studies of adolescents and adults with substance abuse disorder, reported a mean rate of ADHD at 23%. Thus we were puzzled to read that Quinn (1997), along with Wilens and Lineham (1995), concluded that children with ADHD alone were a "negligible risk" for substance abuse. We disagree with this conclusion because we have observed that increasing numbers of ADHD children, representing all three diagnostic subtypes, become involved with drugs and alcohol, sometimes as early as 8 or 9 years old. Huessy and Howell (1985) reported that many ADHD young adults displayed a greater tendency toward alcoholism as adults than a control group of non-ADHD subjects. Of course, there are clear family dimensions related to a child's susceptibility to substance abuse, which we will discuss later. Many of the ADHD inattentive preadolescent children, particularly those entering puberty undiagnosed, become susceptible to a broad range of substance abuse, as well as to mood and anxiety disorders, because of failure in school and conflict with parents. Here the family milieu, including the parental use of alcohol or other intoxicating substances, becomes a clear factor affecting the ADHD child's susceptibility to general substance abuse.

We agree with the report of Wilens and Lineham (1995), who state that the presence of ADHD through adolescence and adulthood increases the risk of substance abuse. Similarly, other studies have reported that the presence of a conduct disorder with ADHD may increase the potential for substance abuse by as much as 20–40% and that the conduct disorder tends to precede substance abuse behaviors (Halikas et al., 1990; Mannuzza et al., 1993).

Learning Disabilities

In our evaluations of potential ADHD children, we explain to parents that a "gray area" often exists between ADHD and learning disability (LD) symptoms and difficulties. We often illustrate this point by drawing a line on a piece of paper to represent a continuum and place ADHD toward the middle and LD toward the end. This is helpful in explaining to parents how there can be an overlap in the symptoms of these disorders. Many ADHD children, but certainly not all, have diagnosable LD problems. Similarly, only a portion of LD children display ADHD symptoms. Barkley (1990a) estimated that as many as 40% of ADHD children may display LD symptoms. This overlap of symptoms is often very confusing to parents, particularly when specific data from testing their child are not yet available, because the criteria for qualifying a child for educational LD services may vary widely, even between neighboring school districts. (We will discuss this issue in Chapter 2.)

LD is typically defined when a "severe discrepancy" exists between a student's cognitive abilities, measured by an IQ test, and her or his actual academic performance, measured by achievement tests. This discrepancy can also be described as the difference between a child's *expected* and *actual* achievement levels. Discrepancy is defined as one and a half to two standard deviations between the two measures (see Heath & Kush, 1991, for a more comprehensive discussion of the determination of LD). The DSM-IV (American Psychiatric Association, 1994) criteria for diagnosing LD involves recognition that the difficulties "interfere with academic achievement or activities of daily living." Specific learning disorders are defined in reading, mathematics, and written expression. It is important for the clinician unfamiliar with LD patterns to recognize that the features of LD can be quite varied, ranging from perceptual, verbal, and motor difficulties to academic, behavioral, and social dysfunctions (Culbertson & Silovsky, 1996).

Barkley (1990a) reported that from 19 to 26% of ADHD children display LD problems, specifically in the areas of math, reading, and spelling. Carlson (1986) reported that in an outpatient clinic population 46% of ADHD "school referrals" had also been diagnosed with an LD. In an earlier study, Carlson and associates (1986) compared groups of grade school children with ADHD, both with and without hyperactivity, with a control group. They reported that the ADHD group with hyperactivity displayed significantly lower Verbal IQ scores and performed more poorly on visual matching tasks than the ADHD group without hyperactivity. Both ADHD groups achieved poorer scores than the control group in spelling and reading. The overall differences between the two ADHD groups were less than they had predicted.

Quinn (1997) discussed this area of LD more broadly under "cognitive deficits." She reported that ADHD children typically display difficulties with problem-solving skills and memory in free-recall situations. Seidman and associates (1995) reported that ADHD students with comorbid LD, ages 9 to 20 years old, demonstrated "reduced motor dominance" and extremely slow reading speeds. They also suggested that a child's performance in these areas may also be affected by family dynamics.

Other Associated Disorders

Two less serious comorbid conditions are sleep disorders and eczema. *Sleep disorders*, a common concern as a potential side effect when ADHD children are taking stimulant medications, are often reported by parents. However, Ball and Koloian (1995) note that "research has been inconclusive" with regard to the effects of stimulant medication on sleep patterns in ADHD children. These authors did report that even though research has not consistently supported differences in sleep disorder patterns between ADHD and non-ADHD children, the parents of ADHD children consistently observe and report the presence of significant sleep disturbance in their children.

A German study (Roth et al., 1991) identified a significantly high incidence of ADHD symptoms in a group of 81 children with *eczema*. These children showed poor performance in attentional capacity and inhibitory functions. The authors suggested a "common predisposing factor" for eczema and ADHD. However, a study by McGee and associates (1993) found no support for the association between ADHD and the presence of allergic disorders such as eczema, asthma, rhinitis, or urticaria in the children studied.

THE DIAGNOSIS OF ADHD IN ADULTS

Despite the extensive research conducted on childhood ADHD, little research has been directed toward understanding and describing the features of ADHD in adults. Even in the clinical setting we suspect that the majority of adults who have underlying ADHD but who present other disorders as their complaint will never be diagnosed with ADHD. Lomas (1995), in a response to concerns regarding the dangers of overdiagnosing ADHD in adults, suggested that most psychiatrists rarely "consider, detect, or treat" adults with ADHD.

In our practices, we consistently find that the manner in which ADHD is first identified in adults is during consultation sessions with parents regarding the evaluation and diagnosis of their child for ADHD. Often we will notice that one parent looks uncomfortable or is squirming in her or his seat as we describe the child's symptoms. Occasionally one parent will get an "odd but knowing" look on her or his face and stare at the partner. Sometimes one parent will blurt out, "It sounds like you're talking about *me* as a child." Or sometimes the other parent will say, either sympathetically or blamingly, "All this sounds like *you!* I always told you that you and Billy were *just alike.*"

To familiarize the clinician with the ADHD diagnosis in adults, we will discuss the following issues:

- How ADHD symptoms continue from childhood into adulthood.
- The incidence of ADHD in adults (epidemiology).
- A critique of the DSM-IV diagnostic criteria for adults and a review of alternate ADHD adult diagnostic criteria.
- The range of ADHD adult symptoms.
- The occurrence of other psychiatric disorders in ADHD adults (comorbidity).

Diagnosis

Early studies estimated that 30–50% of children diagnosed with ADHD would carry the ADHD symptoms into their adult lives (Gittelman et al., 1985; Mannuzza et al., 1991, 1993; Weiss et al., 1985). As we have noted, considerably less attention has been given to ADHD adults in the general literature (Spencer et al., 1994). Quinn (1997) estimated an incidence of ADHD among adults at 40–50% of those who had childhood symptoms, and of these she suggested that 10–15% may display "severe symptoms." We believe that these estimates are quite low and that they will be increased considerably when further research is completed.

The DSM-III (American Psychiatric Association, 1987) only alluded to the potential "persistence" of ADHD in adults who, if diagnosed at all, were placed in the residual subtype category. For all practical purposes, the DSM-IV (American Psychiatric Association, 1994) has not further addressed the existence of the disorder in adults. While it mentions differential ADHD symptoms for "adolescence and adults," it fails to aid clinicians by defining more specific differential criteria. In fact, both diagnostic manuals err in assuming that the ADHD adult symptomatology can be accounted for by the criteria intended for children. In many respects this error of generalization is made with regard to adolescent symptomatology as well.

Wender (1995), a prominent researcher in adult ADHD, critiqued the DSM-III's failure to address adult ADHD or to offer differential criteria. He challenged the assumption that ADHD simply disappears after childhood or adolescence, arguing that it "persists but changes in form." He also pointed out that the use of the "residual type" classification was a misnomer in that it implied that the disorder persisted despite partial recovery. We concur with his view that it is more accurate to assume that ADHD in adults is a "continuation" of the same disorder of childhood. He also believes that many of the childhood symptoms "persist without diminution" in adulthood but are modified by age-related coping and accommodating skills. Contending that many of the criteria used for diagnosing children are irrelevant for diagnosing adults, he cites the criteria from the DSM-III, "sticking to play" and "difficulty awaiting turn in games," to illustrate their utter irrelevancy in diagnosing a "45-year-old professor of comparative literature with ADHD."

Wender's early clinical work (Wender, 1985; Wender, Reimherr, & Wood, 1981) led to the development of what he called the "Utah diagnostic criteria for adult ADHD." His suggested criteria included the recognition of both historic childhood symptoms and presenting adult behaviors. The childhood symptoms are consistent with the general ones we have described previously, that is, inattention, impulsivity, restlessness. In addition to the typical adult symptoms of inattention and hyperactivity, he suggested the presence of other symptoms such as impulsivity, difficulty completing tasks, poor organization, and an intolerance of stress. In his current criteria (Wender, 1995), he defined the presence of both motor and attentional symptoms. Hallowell and Ratey (1994) have also suggested more relevant criteria for ADHD

adults, which include underachievement, poor organization, procrastination, incompletion of tasks, distractibility, impulsivity/impatience,
restlessness, mood swings, insecurity/poor self-esteem, worrying, and
an intolerance to boredom/search for stimulation. We have combined
these lists of criteria in Table 1.3, which can serve as a practical screening tool for adults and their spouses to review together as a general
checklist. It is always important to get observations and feedback from
the spouse or other significant adults in the adult patient's life in order
to corroborate symptoms and behaviors. Often ADHD adults are not
aware of the range of difficult behaviors that may be present in their
relationships.

Cantwell (1996) summarized the research findings regarding the
persistence of childhood ADHD into adult life: "In the past it was
believed that all children with ADD 'outgrew their problem.' This
'outgrowing' was supposed to occur with puberty. We now know
from prospective studies that this is not true" (p. 983). Earlier Cantwell
(1985) had suggested three outcome categories and had estimated the
proportional relationships among them: in 30% of adult subjects the
ADHD symptoms simply disappear in their young adult years; in 40%
the childhood symptoms continue into adult life with associated social
and emotional difficulties; and in 30% the childhood symptoms continue in association with more serious psychopathology, including
alcoholism, drug abuse, and antisocial behaviors.

TABLE 1.3. Comprehensive List of Adult ADHD Symptoms

 1. Hyperactivity/restlessness
 2. Impatience
 3. Intolerance of boredom
 4. Search for high stimulation
 5. Affective lability/mood swings
 6. Hot temper
 7. Stress intolerance
 8. Tendency to worry
 9. Insecurity
10. Poor self-esteem
11. Impulsivity
12. Impaired concentration/distractibility
13. Inability to complete tasks
14. Disorganization
15. Underachievement
16. Procrastination
17. Tendency toward addictive behavior

Note. Symptoms compiled from Hallowell and Ratey (1994) and Wender (1995).

The Range of Adult Symptoms

Adult symptoms of ADHD adults appear as in childhood, though often modified by the differences in age, milieu, and relationships. Certainly, *attention* difficulties may continue into adulthood, but they are not identified as frequently as stressors since the adults are no longer confined in school where the associated difficulties are more readily observed. In addition, some of these adults may have been fortunate to have selected occupations that do not require great attention to details (Wender, 1995). However, because of the presence of attention problems, many adults will report having dropped out of college or technical schools, may express feelings that they are "dumb" or failures compared to their siblings, or may have poor employment histories and/or frequent job changes. Mannuzza and colleagues (1997) periodically interviewed children who had been diagnosed with ADHD as they grew into young adults (24 years old). They noted that, in comparison with a control group, these ADHD adults reported significantly less formal schooling and lower rankings in their occupational positions than the non-ADHD adults.

Poor *short-term memory*, related to the attention problems of childhood, is often a clear and continuing problem for ADHD adults. The inability to remember simple tasks and instructions creates a maddening response from family members, friends, coworkers, and employers. Many adults report forgetting such activities as scheduled meetings or deadlines at work, times to meet spouses or pick up children, or instructions to buy grocery items on the way home from work. We will discuss later how these symptoms can dramatically affect marital dynamics (Chapter 8). Many spouses of ADHD adults often tell us that they have become the "keeper of details" and of schedules for their partners, serving essentially as their memory bank.

Hyperactivity certainly continues into adulthood, though by late adolescence it often begins to modify into an ongoing *restlessness*, a need to *keep moving and busy*, and difficulty *sitting still* when involved in nonstimulating activities. One 40-year-old professional male, as he understood more about the role of ADHD in his life, wept because he finally recognized, and regretted, the "lost years" when he had been unable to *sit still* to read or play with his young children.

This symptom becomes a "two-edged sword" for many adults. Their energy and need for movement can serve many ADHD adults well in certain careers because of the intensity and hyperfocusing that they can put into accomplishing some tasks, particularly in short periods of time. These might include work areas such as corporate decision making, hospital emergency room work, or piloting jet fighters. However, on the negative side, this restless energy diminishes opportunities for communication and intimacy for ADHD adults with both their partners and their children.

While *impulsivity* may be seen as cute or endearing in young children, it has few positive meanings in adult life. For ADHD adults it can often disrupt everyday job responsibilities in the form of poor decision making and/or rash responses in communications and interactions. Some ADHD adults will make sudden decisions to purchase expensive, and often unnecessary, items without consulting with their spouses. Others may make quick reactive comments that may be perceived as harsh, critical, or demeaning by their partner. This trait can create chronically poor interpersonal skills, both in the family and in the work setting. Spouses often perceive this trait as "self-destructive" for their partners, even when they learn that it is tied to the cluster of ADHD symptoms. Of all the ADHD symptoms in adulthood, this may be the most destructive to ongoing interpersonal relationships.

The *disorganization* that resulted in messy rooms and lost assignments in childhood and adolescence can continue to undermine the ADHD adult in both work and personal contexts. For example, the inability to prepare reports in a neat and timely manner, or even keeping one's personal checkbook balanced or keeping tax records, can become a burden for the ADHD adult, not to mention prompt severe reciprocal reactions from their partners and employers.

One of our clients, a 42-year-old man, had worked for about 10 years on an assembly line at a manufacturing company that produced electronic components. One day his employer, recognizing that he had high levels of energy, intensity, and gregariousness, suggested that these personal resources might be better used in the sales field. After a few weeks of training he was sent "on the road" for this first national sales trip. When he returned 2 weeks later, he had, quite remarkably, closed eight out of ten deals worth nearly a half-million dollars for his company. However, during his travels he had lost two of the eight orders; intermingled three of the other orders, such that it was not clear what amounts of the product each of the companies had ordered; and failed to take adequate notes on several specifications.

Fortunately, his boss chose to focus on his strong points and to accommodate his weak points. He made him the first salesperson in the company to have his own laptop computer, a modem, and direct access to a secretary at the home office. Following each deal, he would ask to use a free office to work in (or sometimes simply sit in the lobbies of the office buildings) and immediately record the sale and send the order online back to his company. His salary was in the six-figure bracket when he was referred for marital therapy because his third wife had announced that she would divorce him if he did not get some help for his restlessness, temper, and irritability. He was diagnosed with ADHD. The stimulant medication was so effective in reducing his level of intensity and impulsivity at home that his wife was eager to participate in marital therapy and they made good progress.

Wender (1995) identified the continuation of *affective lability* in ADHD adults as evidenced in sudden mood shifts based on either internal causes or external triggers. The duration of this response is often only minutes or hours, unlike the symptoms of other mood disorders. He reported that many ADHD adults report more "down" than "up" moods in adulthood as compared to their childhoods. However, in our practices we see many ADHD adults who continue to seek stimulation through risky or exciting activities. For example, a 50-year-old depressive ADHD man reported that he was "burned out," that in the past 5 years he had "done it all—white water rafting, rock climbing, flying a stunt plane, hunting in Africa, and parasailing." He had recently recovered from a broken pelvis and leg from a misadventure in the latter pursuit. Another 48-year-old ADHD man severely broke an ankle and a leg when his skydiving parachute failed to open fully on descent.

Patterns of Comorbidity

While the work of identifying differential symptomatic criteria for ADHD adults remains limited, a growing literature attempts to clarify the patterns of *psychiatric comorbidity* that exist in this population. Administering the Minnesota Multiphasic Personality Inventory (MMPI) to ADHD adults, Holdnack and associates (1994) reported that the subjects displayed "mild to moderate" degrees of general psychopathology with multiple scale elevations. Shekim and associates (1990), who studied a group of ADHD adults, ages 19–65, reported comorbid diagnoses of generalized anxiety disorder (53%), alcohol abuse or dependence (34%), drug abuse (30%), dysthymic disorder (25%), and cyclothymic disorder (25%), with *only 12% of the ADHD population displaying no comorbid diagnoses.* Similarly, Tzelepis and associates (1994), in a study of self-referred ADHD adults (81.5% were males), reported the following comorbid conditions: major depression (29%), dysthymia (19%), anxiety disorders (25%; social phobia was the most common, at 11% of the total population), alcohol abuse and dependency (38%), and drug abuse and dependency (26)%. Biederman and his colleagues (1993) reported major depression in 31% of referred ADHD adults and a high rate of depression in the relatives of these ADHD adults: 17% of nonreferred relatives and 29% of nonreferred children in the family as compared to a rate of only 5% in a control group.

Wilens and Lineham (1995) and Wilens and associates (1995b) reported that ADHD in adults typically occurs in conjunction with comorbid disorders of substance abuse as well as mood, anxiety, personality, and learning disorders. They stated that ADHD adults experience a variety of failures in life that lead to a sense of "demoralization and low self-esteem." Other common traits mentioned include stubbornness, procrastination, poor organizational skills, and conflicted relationships with peers, spouses, and authority figures.

An interesting longitudinal study of two ADHD adults compared their life experiences from the period of their original diagnosis at ages 9 and 11 with a follow-up at age 21 (Kramer, 1986). Their histories were fairly consistent except that the subject who displayed more aggression as a child displayed more aggression and participated in more antisocial behavior as an adolescent and as an adult.

Most studies have reported that the familiar comorbid behavioral patterns in childhood ADHD of *conduct, moods, and anxiety disorders* persist into adulthood (Anderson et al., 1987; Cantwell, 1985; Cantwell & Baker, 1989; Gittelman et al., 1985; Mannuzza et al., 1991; Weiss et al., 1985). Biederman and associates (1993) reported that ADHD adults, as compared to a control group, displayed significantly higher rates of *antisocial personality disorder, conduct disorder, oppositional defiant disorder, substance abuse, anxiety disorder, enuresis, stuttering, and speech and language disorders.* To understand the potential of continuing symptoms of conduct disorders in adults, Wender (1995) suggested more caution, citing the need for further research to identify a potential overlap with adult ADHD, conduct disorders, and antisocial personality disorder. Biederman and associates (1993) also compared these adults with a group of ADHD children and found that the children displayed higher rates of oppositional defiant disorder, while the adults displayed higher rates of conduct disorder, substance abuse, anxiety, and stuttering disorders. Carlson and associates (1987) reported a "strong correlation" between "pathological gambling" in adults and histories of ADHD in childhood.

The challenges and difficulties in recognizing the potential for dual diagnoses in ADHD adults have been noted by Schubiner and associations (1995) and Wilens and associates (1995b).

Cognitive disabilities and learning disorders identified in ADHD children have been found to persist into adulthood. An early study (Hopkins et al., 1979) reported that ADHD adults had difficulty selecting from complex relevant stimuli and were more easily distracted by irrelevant stimuli. These adults also had difficulty controlling incorrect verbal statements. Biederman and associates (1993), when comparing ADHD adults with a control group, found that the former displayed significantly lower Full-Scale IQ and freedom-from-distractibility scores, as well as lower scores in vocabulary, block design, digit symbol, arithmetic, and reading. When further compared to a group of ADHD children, the ADHD adults displayed lower block design scores, while the children displayed lower scores in vocabulary, digit span, and freedom from distractibility. Biederman et al. concluded that these cognitive deficits of childhood clearly continue into adulthood.

Holdnack and associates (1995) reported that ADHD adult males, as compared to an adult male control group, displayed slower psychomotor speed, poorer memory with less acquired information and inconsistent semantic clustering, and retroactive interference and item recall inconsistency with overall slower cognitive processing. A retrospective study of ADHD males in their mid-20s reported that, as compared to a non-ADHD control group, the ADHD adults displayed significantly poorer spelling, math, and reading comprehension skills (Claude & Firestone, 1995). Wender (1995) reported that typical symptoms for ADHD adults often include dyslexia and reading disorders. He also observed that arithmetic difficulties often do not affect higher level mathematical abstract reasoning, such as is used in calculus. For example, an ADHD scientist or engineer may conduct complex experiments but make simple arithmetic errors and have difficulty balancing her or his checkbook.

Drug and alcohol abuse occur frequently in populations of ADHD adults (Eyre et al., 1982; Rounsaville, 1993; Wood et al., 1983). However, we have observed that many adults diagnosed and treated for substance abuse disorders have rarely been recognized as also having ADHD. Schubiner and Tzelepis (1996) studied a large sample of 700 substance-abusing adults and found that 25% met the DSM-III-R (American Psychiatric Association, 1987) criteria for ADHD, and 70% of these were males. This comorbidity pattern was associated with a higher incidence of traffic violations, major depression, and antisocial personality disorder for these adults. Biederman and associates (1995b) compared a group of ADHD adults with an adult control group and reported a significantly higher risk of psychoactive substance abuse among the ADHD group (52–77%). While they found little differences in the rate of alcohol-related disorders, they did report that the ADHD group had higher rates of drug and drug-plus-alcohol disorders and that the ADHD significantly increased the risk of the substance abuse disorders independent of comorbid psychiatric disorders. Schubiner and Tzelepis (1996) reported that the most prominently abused substance by ADHD adults was alcohol, not cocaine, as has often been assumed.

The incidence of substance abuse among ADHD adults has been reported at the following rates: *alcohol dependence*, 23%; *marijuana*, 9%; *cocaine*, 6%; *polydrug*, 5% (Tzelepis et al., 1994). Wilens and associates (1994) estimated similar substance abuse rates for ADHD adults, ranging from *17–45% for alcohol abuse and dependence and 9–30% for drug abuse and drug dependence*. Schubiner and associates (1995) studied substance abuse in several ADHD adult males and found patterns that supported the self-medication theory in the use of alcohol. They also reported the successful use of psychostimulants in treating these substance-abusing ADHD adults, who were alcohol- and drug-free 2 to 3 years following the onset of treatment. However, Wilens and associates (1994) recommended that active substance-abusing adults be "stabilized" before any pharmacologic treatment for ADHD is begun.

The common comorbid psychiatric disorders for adults are listed in Table 1.4.

In the following chapter, we will discuss the timing of the ADHD diagnosis and dilemmas related to the differential diagnosis.

TABLE 1.4. Psychiatric Disorders Comorbid with Adult ADHD

1. Anxiety disorders	6. Personality disorders
2. Substance abuse/dependence	7. Learning disabilities
3. Depression	8. Conduct disorder
4. Dysthymia	9. Oppositional defiant disorder
5. Cyclothymic disorder	10. Speech and language disorders

2

The Clinical Evaluation: Diagnosing, Consultation, Testing, and the Use of Medication

The evaluation of ADHD is a critical clinical process and, in most cases, relies heavily upon thorough history taking, interaction with family sources to obtain corroborating information, the utilization of psychometric data, and medical evaluation for the use of stimulant or other medications in treatment. We emphasize the benefits of multidisciplinary teams working together in the evaluation and treatment of ADHD; realistically, a single clinician is not equipped by training to conduct the entire evaluation. We will discuss the value of the interdisciplinary team in the next chapter. However, it is important for the primary therapist, who will be working with the ADHD individual and his or her family, to understand the ingredients of the overall process and to make referrals when appropriate.

In this chapter we will discuss the important practical aspects of:

1. Recognizing the "red flags" that indicate the clusters of ADHD symptoms that may occur in children, adolescents, and adults who may never have been in treatment or who may be in therapy for one or more of the previously identified comorbid disorders.
2. Documenting the historical development of symptoms consistent with the diagnostic criteria.
3. Identifying the specific symptomatology consistent with the DSM-IV criteria.
4. Determining the influence of the ADHD symptoms on an

individual's overall development, as well as concurrent parent–child and sibling interactions.

5. Determining the influence of the symptoms on an adult's family and marital experiences.
6. Identifying specific dysfunctions resulting from the ADHD symptoms in the child's school and social functioning.
7. Identifying specific dysfunctions resulting from the symptoms in the adult's educational and career functioning.
8. Determining the need for accommodations in educational or employment settings.
9. Determining the need for psychoeducational testing.
10. Determining the need for psychopharmacological evaluation.
11. Developing an effective treatment plan for the ADHD individual, his or her family, and his or her educational and/or work setting.
12. Determining the need for consultation with other clinical and/or education professionals involved with the family.

MAKING A DIFFERENTIAL DIAGNOSIS WITH ADHD

The differential aspects of an ADHD diagnosis are particularly difficult for clinicians because of the high incidence and frequency of many comorbid disorders. Although there is some concern that these additional psychiatric disorders may be "mistakenly" identified as ADHD (AACAP, 1997), we are more concerned that ADHD symptoms are often camouflaged by comorbid disorders or simply go unrecognized by many clinicians. Consequently, many individuals with ADHD may never be diagnosed, or at least not diagnosed in a timely fashion.

The importance of the differential diagnosis is heightened by the fact that *most children and adults present for therapy with the comorbid symptoms and not with ADHD.* Clinicians, like teachers, encounter the ongoing dilemma of distinguishing the symptoms of oppositional and conduct disorders from those of ADHD. It is even more of a challenge in grade school settings to recognize the existence of inattentive-type ADHD children, who are often viewed by their teachers as bright and capable but "lazy and unmotivated." These children's intellectual resources often mask the ADHD symptoms (Bar-Josef et al., 1995). In addition to being alert for the potential presence of psychiatric disorders, clinicians must also screen clinical populations of children and adolescents carefully for (1) family dynamics (such as abuse, conflict, and divorce) that may either promote similar symptoms that do not arise from ADHD or that may camouflage the underlying ADHD symptoms, and (2) learning disabilities (LD) that can be either independent of ADHD or associated with it.

For clinicians working in agencies or private settings, the dilemmas are similar because the referring problems for most ADHD children and adults will identify the comorbid conditions more often than the explicit ADHD symptoms. Clinicians wishing to become more skilled in this area of practice will need to learn to recognize the red flags of ADHD that are typically embedded in the individual's everyday struggles with life and the ongoing conflicts that are present in his or her family, peer, and social relationships. The clinician's observational and diagnostic skills will be challenged in this role.

The importance of differential diagnosis with ADHD has been addressed throughout the literature. Quinn (1997) posed the following question: "But do some of these [ADHD] children simply represent a state of hyperarousal and hypervigilance which results in overanxiety or do they represent a true anxiety disorder? The clinician will need to answer this question on a case by case basis" (p. 215). Cantwell (1996) summarized the task: "The differential diagnosis must rule out the presence of other psychiatric disorders, developmental disorders, and medical and neurological disorders and determine whether these are comorbid or whether they are mimicking an ADD syndrome" (p. 981). Similarly, Gadow and Sprafkin (1996) observed: "Because emotional and behavioral disorders generally respond best to certain types of treatment and the presence of multiple problems greatly complicates clinical management, it is very important to accurately determine the type of disability a youngster is experiencing" (p. 1).

One of the most difficult challenges of differential diagnosis for the clinician is that of distinguishing between ADHD and the presence of a *bipolar disorder*. Strober (1996), who has followed 54 children and adolescents with bipolar disorders over a 5-year period, reported that misdiagnosing bipolar children as having ADHD delayed their proper treatment—often until adulthood. He observed that these bipolar children displayed bursts of irritability, emotional lability, affective dysregulation, anxiety, and hyperactivity or hypomania. He believed that it is the presence of "affect storms"—intense verbosity and hyperactivity seen in early onset bipolar illness—that often leads to the misdiagnosis of ADHD. He offered the helpful differentiation that these bipolar children and adolescents displayed more sustained mood shifts, more frantic goal-directed behaviors, and a greater susceptibility to weepiness, suspiciousness, and anxiety. He also observed that many adults with bipolar disorder recalled being diagnosed with ADHD as children or adolescents and medicated with stimulants.

Popper (1989), a child psychopharmacologist, has indicated that these two disorders, ADHD and bipolar disorder, are very hard to differentiate in children and adolescents because of their many similar characteristics: impulsivity, inattention, hyperactivity, physical energy, behavioral and emotional lability, frequent comorbid conduct disorder, frequent oppositional defiant disorder, learning problems, cognitive "looseness," motor restlessness during sleep, and family histories of mood disorders. He summarized the primary differentiating factors between these two disorders as follows:

> ADHD children, in general, display no psychotic symptoms, whereas bipolar children exhibit more gross distortion in perceptions of reality or in affective experiences, such as paranoid-like thinking or sadistic impulses.
>
> ADHD children can be destructive and do break things through carelessness, but bipolar children display more severe temper tantrums involving anger and manic qualities.
>
> ADHD children's anger usually subsides within 20 to 30 minutes, whereas bipolar children's anger may continue for several hours, during which they may display more regression than the child with ADHD, often to the point of losing physical, cognitive, and linguistic functions.
>
> ADHD children's tantrums are often triggered by sensory or affective overstimulation, whereas bipolar children's tantrums are typically triggered by limit setting.
>
> ADHD children are often oblivious to danger and power struggles, whereas bipolar children seem to enjoy both.
>
> Bipolar children, unlike ADHD children, display more dysphoria and irritability and greater fluctuations in appetite and body weight.

Popper also noted that these disorders can coexist in the same child and that stimulants can be used in combination with lithium to treat the comorbid disorders simultaneously. He suggested that when ADHD symptoms persist after lithium has controlled the bipolar symptoms, the additional diagnosis of ADHD and a "lithium-plus-stimulant treatment" is appropriate.

Reiff and associates (1993) have recommended that a thorough evaluation for ADHD children and adolescents should include the following:

1. An interview with parents to obtain developmental, medical, and social histories.

2. An interview with the child to determine developmental levels and symptomatology.
3. A medical evaluation for health, sensory, and neurological screening.
4. A cognitive assessment.
5. Parent and teacher rating scales.
6. Speech, language, and motor skills assessments.

Some therapists may feel overwhelmed at the prospect of being involved in such an extensive evaluation. Many may feel that they do not have the training to complete this type of evaluation on their own. The benefits of working in an interdisciplinary network of other professionals will become apparent as we discuss evaluation and treatment issues in this and the following chapter.

A NOTE ABOUT THE TIMING
OF THE INITIAL DIAGNOSIS

It is important for therapists to recognize the wide variability that exists in the timing of the initial ADHD diagnosis for children, adolescents, and adults We believe that the majority of individuals with ADHD *have not been, and may never be, diagnosed during their school years.* Perhaps less than one-quarter of the ADHD population will be diagnosed before or during their early years of grade school. We hope that, as a result of the increased professional and parental awareness of the disorder, this sad situation will begin to change for the present generation of children entering school. However, we would estimate that as many as 50% of undiagnosed ADHD individuals will carry their personal struggles with the disorder into their young adult lives, their marriages, and eventually into their own parenting roles without any awareness of the effects of the disorder or its potential for treatment. Unfortunately, the ADHD diagnosis is still somewhat "hit or miss," depending on the personal awareness of a teacher, a pediatrician, a therapist, a parent, or some other concerned individual.

We see many ADHD individuals—children, adolescents, and adults—who have been in psychotherapy for a variety of disorders for many years but whose therapists did not have an awareness of, or the skills to recognize, the existing cluster of ADHD symptoms. Many of the children's presenting symptoms were accepted at face value by their therapists, who failed to consider the history and/or underlying behaviors that are red flags for ADHD. We often work with children and adolescents who are failing academically and whose teachers, school counselors, and school psychologists have not recognized their ADHD symptoms. We also see children and adolescents who have been in serious behavioral difficulties in their schools (some of whom have been threatened with expulsion) where ADHD symptoms as causative factors have been ignored or even overtly denied by professionals. We commonly hear the complaint from parents that a teacher or school counselor had dismissed the notion of their child having ADHD when the parent had raised the possibility, perhaps years ago, after reading or hearing something pertaining to the disorder.

We also see many children falling behind academically in basic reading and mathematics skills by the fifth and sixth grades who continue to be labeled by teachers and school counselors as lazy, underachieving, or unmotivated. Many teachers and school counselors simply do not have the training or the time to ask the broader questions regarding why a child of at least average and perhaps above-average intelligence is struggling and failing. We know a single parent who was recently told by a grade school principal that because her fifth-grade son was lying about his lost assignments and incomplete homework, the mother should be concerned that he will become a "psychopath" by the time he is 14 years old. The child was diagnosed, independently of the school, with ADHD. However, at a meeting with the parent, teachers, and the principal where the psychometric results were presented by one of the authors (CAE), the principal continued to maintain that the child was just lazy and needed more guidance from the mother.

Recently, one of the authors (CAE) evaluated a 13-year-old girl who had just begun middle school. She was referred for fighting with her peers and for confrontations with her teachers. A brief telephone consultation with one of her teachers revealed that she had already been labeled, after just 2 months in this new school, as a troublemaker and even a dangerous child. Her school counselor said, "I cannot understand how she made it to seventh grade because she can hardly read." This school counselor had interviewed the student on five occasions about her behavior problems and academic failures and reported to the vice-principal and to the parents that the student had very limited intellectual resources.

Despite her pronouncement, the counselor never offered to have the student tested to determine more specifically her learning potential. As some school personnel often do, perhaps understandably, this counselor responded more to the dramatic and occasionally threatening behaviors of the student and did not examine more objectively the broader picture of the student's overall struggles. Even when one of the authors (CAE) became involved, the school authorities still refused to test the student because they felt that she was primarily a behavioral problem and the parents should get her into therapy. We had the student tested privately. The test data confirmed the ADHD diagnosis. Moreover, her Full-Scale score on the WISC-III was 138!

We encounter similar case situations everyday in our practices. Their frequent occurrence only underlines the importance of looking beyond the labels placed on children and adolescents by teachers or other school personnel. It is important for the clinician to recognize the cluster of ADHD symptoms that may be present in an individual's social and educational histories, and build a collection of clinical data to either support or rule out the diagnosis of ADHD. Unlike the symptoms of many other psychiatric disorders, the ADHD symptoms may be present from the earliest years of the patient's life—as will the reciprocal responses in the family system.

ADHD children who are quite hyperactive may be identified as early as 2 to 3 years of age, while others may not be recognized until they reach kindergarten or first grade. Some ADHD children, predominantly inattentive type, may not be diagnosed until they make the difficult transition to middle school as young adolescents. In fact, we believe that the majority of these inattentive children and adolescents may never be diagnosed during their educational years.

PSYCHOEDUCATIONAL TESTING AND PROCEDURES

Even when the therapist working with ADHD individuals and families is not trained to conduct psychoeducational testing, he or she must be familiar with the testing resources, procedures, and use of data. Unlike other general mental health diagnoses, which rely primarily on history and clinical observations, the ADHD diagnosis should also be supported by psychometric data. In addition, these data provide the therapist with specific resources to guide both educational and clinical interventions.

The public schools are mandated by federal and state laws to screen students for learning disabilities (LD). If a child is actually failing a number of subjects or falling blatantly behind in certain basic learning skills, such as reading or math, the school will do testing to evaluate whether the child is learning-disabled. Often this is determined by looking at the discrepancy between the child's actual performance in school and her or his ability as measured by a variety of testing instruments. However, we have learned that in the absence of an outside professional or advocate working with the parents of an

ADHD child, educators may simply tell parents that their child tested fine: "His test results showed that his IQ is average and the other tests showed that he just needed to work harder on his math. *He does not qualify for special education services."*

This cursory testing profile will fit a large percentage of ADHD students who do, indeed, have average or high IQ's and who therefore will not "qualify" for or "need" special education services. Of course, the testing may help identify some of the nearly 50% of ADHD students estimated to display LD (Shaywitz & Shaywitz, 1988). However, though they may test for LD, many school personnel fail to evaluate for, or recognize, the underlying symptoms of ADHD unless the disorder is quite severe. Some school evaluators will overlook or fail to recognize ADHD symptoms and patterns in the testing even when specifically asked to consider their presence by an outside professional or a parent. Certainly, many school districts have limited funding and resources for testing. However, we still find some school administrators who are reluctant to accept an ADHD diagnosis as having validity. One assistant principal recently stated: "How can you be so sure that he has ADHD? No one even knows if that is a legitimate disorder!"

School policies with regard to testing and evaluating will vary according to state and even community guidelines. For example, one managed care group in a western state, from which we occasionally seek testing approval, invariably lectures us on the fact that we are asking them to reimburse for ADHD testing: "This kind of testing should be completed in the schools, not by mental health professionals. We never have to pay for it in our community because the schools always do it." However, in our community, school administrators and school psychologists make it quite clear that they neither test for nor diagnose ADHD. Their position is that ADHD is a psychiatric disorder and therefore not within their area of expertise. As we have stated, they are required to evaluate students and rule out the possibility of a learning disorder. In the process of this evaluation they will undoubtedly collect data that will be indicative of ADHD if it is present.

Therefore, depending on the policies within one's community, turning to private testing may be necessary. The referral for this testing needs to be made carefully. Another managed care group that we occasionally work with will pay for testing for ADHD on their own terms. This has meant referral to clinical psychologists who complete a broad and expensive ($900–$1,200) battery of traditional psychological tests ranging from the MMPI to projective instruments, regardless of the referral question. Even though we have told this managed care group that much of that testing is not only unnecessary but irrelevant to our referral for testing to evaluate for ADHD, they have maintained the position that this was the only testing for which they would pay.

An additional dilemma that we have encountered in working with schools is that even when schools are willing to complete ADHD testing, such testing is not seen as a priority. Many times the testing will be delayed until the next semester or the end of the school year. And, of course, it is typically impossible to obtain testing during the summer months or early in the fall semester. Obviously, if the clinician and parents need testing results to confirm diagnostic issues, which then would affect both therapeutic and perhaps medical interventions, such delay could cost the child further difficulties and a greater loss of learning potential. These issues point to the need for the clinician to be able to refer ADHD families for appropriate testing in a timely manner.

For the clinician working predominantly with ADHD children and adolescents, finding a psychometrist who is experienced in testing for ADHD is essential. We use the term *psychometrist* because it broadly defines the primary role of a testing specialist. These individuals may be special education teachers, school psychologists, or clinical psychologists. The need for such a resource, whether one is a clinician in private practice or working in an agency setting, highlights two dilemmas that both clinicians and parents face in working with school systems. First, as we have indicated, many school districts will not, or cannot, make the diagnosis of ADHD, since it is a psychiatric disorder and not an educational disorder. However, we continue to be appalled by how often parents are told by a classroom teacher or a school counselor that their child *definitely does not have ADHD* and simply needs to work harder or get more assistance from the parents. The more responsive schools, however, will suggest to the parents that they take the child to a pediatrician or a therapist in order to obtain a diagnosis. In addition, many school administrators, and some school psychologists, are not able or willing to allocate their limited testing time and funds for ADHD screening, particularly if the student is getting mostly passing grades. They are also less responsive to testing requests made *just* by a parent unhappy with her or his child's performance in school.

We have worked for nearly 10 years with a clinical psychologist who specializes in psychoeducational testing with children and adolescents. We have found it quite beneficial to be able to refer parents to this colleague to conduct the actual testing. The parents appreciate gaining a second opinion and we can maintain our role in the evaluation and treatment process separate from the testing process. Often only a couple of tests are necessary to support the clinical diagnosis of ADHD. When we refer an individual to our colleague for "ADHD testing," she knows exactly what we are expecting. There is no repetition of extensive history taking because we send her a brief memorandum summarizing the personal, educational, and family history, as well as our own observations, before she sees the child we have referred (see Appendix 2.1 for a sample referral letter). We will also let her know if we are looking for other comorbid mental health concerns, such as depression. She does not need to repeat our screening procedures, so she schedules two 1½-hour sessions for the testing. In the first session she administers the Wechsler Intelligence Scale for Children—III, and in the second, the ability and achievement tests that make up the Woodcock–Johnson Psycho-Educational Battery—Revised. She may administer other tests if we express concern about a comorbid disorder. We also let her know whether we are requesting just a brief summary report for our own interpretive purposes with the parents, or we need a more detailed educational report to submit to the school. She also sends us the specific protocols (testing data) for each of the tests, which aid us in our review and interpretation of the data, as well as in explaining the patterns related to ADHD for the student and her or his parents. These data will also direct us in developing a plan for requesting potential educational accommodations with the school (we will discuss these later) and in developing specific therapeutic interventions.

In seeking a psychometrist with whom to work, we recommend looking for professionals who have worked in educational settings. Certainly, many clinical psychologists are qualified to perform testing. However, our experience is that many psychologists who perform testing as part of a general or forensic practice provide a broad range of traditional psychological tests (e.g., MMPI, TAT, Rorschach, etc.) even when advised that the diagnostic concern is primarily ADHD. As illustrated above, we have found this to be particularly problematic in dealing with certain managed care groups who determine both the "justification" of testing for ADHD and the "psychologist" who can be certified to do the testing. The insurance reimbursement for ADHD testing, as well as for other psychological testing, is quite variable. Technically, the testing that we mentioned for ADHD is *psychoeducational* rather than purely psychological. One large managed care group, from which some of our ADHD families receive services, will only certify for testing for ADHD when we are also looking for other concurrent symptoms, such as depression.

The availability of a qualified and interested psychometrist for ADHD referrals will not only facilitate one's clinical role with the family but also provide a more focused, efficient, and often less expensive testing resource for ADHD families. Many of the families we work with choose to pay out of pocket for private testing rather than go through the often frustrating and time-consuming process of attempting to get either the school or their insurance carrier to pay for it. Sometimes the privacy issue is important to the parents. For example, one father recently told us that he would rather pay for the testing privately because if there were no positive findings to support either an ADHD or LD diagnosis, then it would never appear on his child's records. He worked in a high-security career position and had learned how even insignificant historical events might surface later in the process of obtaining a security clearance.

An Introduction to Specific Testing Instruments and Procedures

Since psychoeducational testing is a central component in the evaluation of ADHD, clinicians working in this area need to be familiar with the primary tests and how to interpret them to parents and ADHD individuals. Most clinicians are exposed to some general aspects of more traditional psychological testing in their education and training. These may include projective tests such as the Rorschach and the Thematic Apperception Test (TAT), the universally recognized Minnesota Multiphasic Personality Inventory (MMPI-2), and perhaps a variety of symptom-specific tests related to anxiety or depression. Psychoeducational testing is clearly different from, and more specialized than, these general psychological testing instruments. It is essential for clinicians working with ADHD individuals to be able to understand the data gained from these tests so that they can be discussed knowledgeably and accurately with both family members and school personnel. Therefore, we will briefly review the tests we have found helpful in this evaluation process and identify the basic components that clinicians need to understand with regard to ADHD.

No single instrument has been developed to assess ADHD directly. The general parent and teacher questionnaires with which clinicians may be familiar are for screening purposes and not for the diagnosis of cognitive processing patterns. Thus the evaluation usually includes several specific psychoeducational instruments, namely, the Wechsler Intelligence Scale for Children—Third Edition (WISC-III), or for adults, the Wechsler Adult Intelligence Scale—Revised (WAIS-R), and more recently the WAIS-III; and the Woodcock–Johnson Psycho-Educational Battery—Revised (WJ-R). These tests may be supported by a variety of rating scales that have been developed to add observations and data from external "informants" such as teachers and parents. In recent years a variety of additional tests have been developed and are still being refined with regard to their validity and reliability in the examination of specific areas of ADHD symptoms, such as distractibility, concentration, and auditory and visual processing (Klee, 1986; Zarski et al., 1987).

The Wechsler Intelligence Scale for Children (WISC-III) and the Wechsler Adult Intelligence Scale (WAIS-III)

These tests, which are utilized respectively for children and adults, are almost universally accepted as reliable measures of an individual's intellectual functioning in what has become known as the "IQ" score. They are utilized in a broad range of psychoeducational testing to establish a baseline for a student's intellectual functioning and potential, which can then be compared to actual academic achievement and classroom grades. Scores from these tests are often used to qualify students at one or the other end of a continuum: as "gifted" or as learning disabled (LD) and in need of special education services.

As part of the psychoeducational assessment of ADHD, the data from these tests (Verbal, Performance, and "Full-Scale" scores) provide both a baseline of the student's intellectual abilities and, through the analysis of the test's subtests, a comparative pattern of strengths and deficits from which important data can be gleaned. For example, a student receiving B's and C's in her classroom work who obtained a Full-Scale IQ of 112, Verbal IQ of 114, and Performance IQ of 110 on the WISC-III would show no red flags, since her school grades and her Full-Scale score (in the "high average" range) are fairly congruent. From these scores, it might be suggested that the student could actually perform at a somewhat higher achievement level with more motivation or more serious work habits.

As a contrasting example, another student has the same WISC-III Full-Scale score of 112 but a 102 Verbal score and a 120 Performance score. Her grades are reported as C's, D's, and an occasional F. Here there are at least two red flags. First, the discrepancy of 18 points between the Verbal and Performance scores is significant. A rule of thumb among practitioners is that any discrepancy over 10 to 12 points between these two scores may raise a concern. This student's performance skills far outweigh her verbal skills, which is often indicative of a functional problem. The second red flag here is that the child's high-average Full-Scale score of 112 should be indicative of grades much better than those reported. At the very least this means that the student is seriously underachieving in school. The broader diagnostic issue here is to identify the etiology of this discrepancy.

After a review of the gross Verbal and Performance scores, the psychometrist reviews the subtest scores in order to identify the individual's pattern of strengths and weaknesses. There are six subtests that make up the Verbal Scale and seven in the Performance Scale. The Verbal scale subtests include Information, Similarities, Arithmetic, Vocabulary, Comprehension, and Digit Span. The Performance scale subtests include Picture Completion, Coding, Picture Arrangement, Block Design, Object Assembly, Symbol Search, and Mazes.

When the therapist receives the testing report and subscale scores, she or he can easily scan the comparative scores in these areas. Many will be within the average range. However, in the latter student's case, several scores stand out because they are only 4 or 5, or borderline. Since the student's Verbal score was only 102, as compared to her Performance score of 120, one would expect to find a lower range of scores among the verbal subtests. The possible red flags for ADHD in general among all the subtests would include below-average scores in such areas as arithmetic, digit span, comprehension, coding, picture arrangement, and block design. In this student's case, the lower scores are in the subtests of Digit Span and Coding or Vocabulary and Comprehension. Her higher scores are in the Performance subtests of Picture Completion, Block Design, and Object Assembly; many of these are above average.

A psychometrist can analyze these subtests to produce summary scores in areas such as Verbal Conceptualization, Perceptual Organization, and Processing Speed. The WISC-III also has a "freedom from distractibility" (FFD) index score that many psychometrists report. It is based on the subtest scores for Arithmetic and Digit Span. However, the reliability of this FFD factor is debated in the literature, most recently by Bernard (1995). Its role was originally defined, with slightly differing technical calculations, by Sattler (1988) and Kaufman (1980).

We have found that once clinicians become familiar with scores on the WISC-III and WAIS-III subtests and understand the overall role of the Performance and Verbal scores, their discussion of the psychometrist's findings with the family becomes considerably easier. If clinicians have limited familiarity with these tests and their interpretation, we recommend that they invite the psychometrist to participate in feedback sessions with the parents. Several such meetings will aid therapists in gaining both confidence and effectiveness in discussing the testing results with families on their own.

The WAIS-III is essentially the same test designed for adult populations. It provides overall data and interpretation similar to those of the WISC-III.

The Woodcock–Johnson
Psycho-Educational Battery—Revised (WJ-R)

The WJ-R is the primary psychoeducational instrument used, often in conjunction with the WISC-III or the WAIS-III, to determine cognitive processing skills and achievement levels. It is comprised of two parts: Tests of Cognitive Ability and Tests of Achievement. Many schools administer only the achievement portions of this test to determine if a student is functioning at grade level. However, our colleagues find that the complete test results must be available in order to evaluate the presence or absence of patterns suggestive of ADHD.

This test is considerably more detailed and complex than the WISC-III/WAIS-III. Thus, clinicians often must rely on the psychometrist to provide a summary evaluation of a student's strengths and deficits. The measurement of students' cognitive functioning by this test identifies their overall broad cognitive abilities. It is based on subtests that measure short-term memory, comprehension-knowledge, visual processing, auditory processing, long-term retrieval, fluid reasoning, and processing speed. Parts of this test are often interesting and occasionally "fun" for students to take. For example, on the Picture Vocabulary subtest the student is shown a variety of pictures and asked to name familiar objects. This section measures both breadth and depth of knowledge *and* the student's verbal communication skills. In a different format, the Listening Comprehension subtest asks the student to listen to a brief audio recording and to verbally supply the missing word in the audio segment.

Deficits in the areas of auditory and visual processing have been associated closely with ADHD symptoms. A central auditory processing disorder appears quite commonly with ADHD and is often responsive to stimulant medications (Gascon et al., 1986; Jerome, 1995; Molt, 1996). In the WJ-R, the "Auditory Processing" cluster measures the student's ability to analyze and synthesize auditory information. The "Incomplete Words" subtest in this cluster is a measure of auditory processing skills; the student is asked to listen to recorded words that are missing one or more phonemes and then is tested to determine whether the words are understood. Similar tests of the Visual Processing cluster measure the student's ability to analyze and synthesize visual stimuli. For example, on the Visual Closure subtest the student is asked to identify pictures of simple objects that have been altered in some manner.

Another area related to the assessment of ADHD is that of "Processing Speed." This cluster of tests measures the student's ability to rapidly perform fairly automatic cognitive tasks when under the pressure of maintaining focused attention. The related "Visual Matching" test asks a student to work quickly and maintain attention while identifying and circling two identical numbers in a sequence of six numbers.

The Tests of Cognitive Ability portion of the WJ-R measures the student's potential for achievement in areas of general knowledge, reading, written language, and mathematics. The Tests of Achievement portion of the test measures actual achievement in areas such as basic and broad reading, mathematics reasoning, basic writing skills, and written expression. These scores in ability and achievement are also compared for discrepancies. The overall results of the WJ-R are reported in percentile and standard scores (which can be compared to IQ scores) and percentile ranks, with the subject's scores defined according to age and grade level. In the case of the student whom we reviewed, her weaknesses were identified by the WISC-III in the verbal areas, and one might expect to see scores in mathematics or calculation at below average levels. The same might also be true with her scores in sound blending and auditory processing. Her scores in visual closure, reading, and visual matching might be at above-average levels.

Harvey and Chernouskas (1995) reported that the results of the WJ-R can be a useful component in the overall diagnostic process for ADHD, but argued that because of the somewhat variable and idiosyncratic nature of specific ADHD symptoms, the WJ-R should not be used in isolation from other measures. They viewed the patterns of cognitive and academic strengths and weaknesses identified by the test as helpful in developing individualized treatment and educational plans. Many ADHD individuals will display, for example, clear auditory processing weaknesses and low processing speeds but high to superior levels of visual processing. Other ADHD individuals may display just the opposite pattern, and some will display weaknesses in both areas. This is why the WJ-R and the WISC-III/WAIS-III are typically administered and evaluated concurrently, and with additional information provided by parent and teacher rating scales.

In addition to the WISC-III/WAIS-III and WJ-R, there has been some limited discussion in the literature of the use of projective instruments in the assessment of ADHD. Costantino and his colleagues (1991) reported that the use of the Tell-Me-A-Story apperception test was useful in evaluating ADHD children because it provided direct observation of subjects' behaviors and provided a mechanism for the scoring of their responses to the details of the stories. Pantle and colleagues (1994) used the Gordon Continuous Performance Test (CPT; Gordon, 1986; Gordon & Metelman, 1988; a computer-based visually interactive measure that we will discuss later) to evaluate the effectiveness of the Rorschach in assessing ADHD subjects' impulsivity. They concluded that certain variables of the Rorschach were reliable in assessing this trait.

The Use of Rating Scales to Screen for ADHD

Beyond these formal psychoeducational tests, a variety of self- and informant-reporting scales have been developed to assist clinicians in gaining additional data from the individuals being evaluated and corroborating sources regarding the presence of ADHD symptoms (see Table 2.1). For young children and grade school-age children, the primary reports are derived from parent and teacher checklists. These scales are not as technically sophisticated as those discussed above. They usually involve a simple listing of statements that reflect the broad range of ADHD symptoms. The lists of these statements are formatted such that a parent and teacher can simply read through and check the items or symptoms that apply. Many of these checklists have

TABLE 2.1. Rating Scales and Checklists

For children

ADD Comprehensive Teacher Rating Scale (ACTeRS; Ullmann et al., 1990)
Attention Deficit Disorders Evaluation Scale (ADDES; McCarney, 1995)
Child Behavior Checklist (Achenbach, 1991)
Child Symptom Inventories (CSI; Gadow & Sprafkin, 1994)
Conners Parent and Teacher Questionnaires (Conners, 1989)
Home and School Situations Questionnaires (Barkley, 1991)

For adolescents

ADD/H Adolescent Self-Report Scale (Conners & Wells, 1985)
ADD/H Adolescent Self-Report Scale—Revised (Vandermay & Robin, 1994)
ANSER Systems Forms (Levine, 1985)
Brown Attention-Deficit Disorder Scales (BADDS; Brown, 1996)

For adults

Adult ADD Questionnaire (Nadeau, 1995)
Attention-Deficit Scales for Adults (ADSA; Triolo, 1996)
Brown Attention-Deficit Disorder Scales (BADDS; Brown, 1995)
Conners Adult ADHD History Form (Conners, 1995)
Copeland Symptom Checklist for Adult Attention Deficit Disorders
    (Copeland, 1994)
Unnamed Checklist (Hallowell & Ratey, 1994)
Wender Utah Rating Scale (Wender, 1995)

been developed to provide reliability, internal consistency, and the ability to accurately identify ADHD populations.

As additional sources of data, these checklists should be viewed as secondary tools to assist in confirming or ruling out the ADHD diagnosis. Some of these popular scales are quite lengthy, such that they can test the motivation of the respondents. For example, the results of a mother's perceptions of her child's behaviors may be highly indicative of the ADHD symptoms. However, the scores on the same scale from a less involved father who does not attempt to answer all the items or from a teacher who fills it out hurriedly during recess break may not provide any support for or consistency with the mother's report. Again, we want to stress that these rating scales provide corroborating information to assist in the diagnosis: *they should not be considered as diagnostic on their own.*

When asked to evaluate a potential ADHD student by a teacher or therapist, many schools will give one of these rating scales to the student's teacher (or to several teachers for a middle or high school student). If the results of these scores do not clearly support criteria for ADHD, the school may refuse to do further testing. However, we have reviewed sets of checklists generated for students by teachers and have found many that were not completed and some where a teacher mechanically checked every item down one column. We know of several pediatricians who routinely send these scales home to parents and to the schools for teachers to complete. The results are often used to support their decisions as to whether or not to prescribe stimulant medications. One physician in our community, who does not work or consult with many therapists, stated that he kept these checklists in his ADHD patients' files so that if he were ever asked for documentation by the medical board regarding his use of stimulants with children, he could "defend" himself. Many of his young patients were never referred for more complete evaluations, and only a few were ever tested further by the schools. Some of his patients undoubtedly could have benefited from the stimulant medications, but they were never formally diagnosed as ADHD in his files because the data from the rating scales did not meet ADHD criteria.

The most common of the rating scales utilized by the schools and some professionals are the Achenbach Child Behavior Checklist (1991) and the Conners Parent and Teacher Questionnaires (1989). Additional ones include the Child Symptom Inventories (CSI) (Gadow & Sprafkin, 1994), the Attention Deficit Disorders Evaluation Scale (ADDES) (McCarney, 1995), the Barkley (1991) Home and School Situations Questionnaires, and the ADD Comprehensive Teacher Rating Scale (ACTeRS; Ullmann, 1985; Ullmann et al., 1984, 1990). Many studies have evaluated the comparative abilities of these instruments in accurately identifying ADHD symptoms. Kuehne and associates (1987), in a comparative study of a variety of instruments with grade school-age children, reported that the Conners Parent and Teacher Questionnaires (1989) accurately discriminated among three matched groups of boys: those with ADHD, those with LD, and a control group. We have used the ACTeRS instrument for several years because it is brief, straightforward, and colorful. It offers separate profiles for girls and boys in areas of attention, hyperactivity, social skills, and oppositional behaviors. We have found that because of its brief and engaging format, we receive more careful and serious responses from teachers. It has been standardized and provides for rapid scoring and interpretation (Ullmann et al., 1984, 1985).

There are self-report rating scales available for adolescents in addition to the parent and teacher reports identified above. The best known of these are the Brown Attention-Deficit Disorder Scale (BADDS; Brown, 1996), the ADD/H Adolescent Self-Report Scale (Conners & Wells, 1985), and the ANSER Systems Forms (Levine, 1985). We have found that a brief, 12-item Likert-type scale adaptation of the Conners and Wells instrument, developed by Vandermay and Robin (1994), is consistently effective in the initial screening of potential ADHD adolescents.

There are a variety of self-report rating scales for adults. Many of these simply list diagnostic criteria from the DSM-IV (American Psychiatric Association, 1994). Others extrapolate from these criteria, using more practical statements of symptomatic behaviors, such as the one presented in Hallowell and Ratey's book (1994), which identifies 20 behavioral items (see Table 1.4 for a summary of some of their items) and suggests that if 15 are answered affirmatively, there is a reasonable concern that ADHD is present. Wender (1995) developed a somewhat more formal 61-item ADHD rating scale for adults, The Wender Utah Rating Scale, and a Targeted Attention-Deficit Disorder Symptoms Rating Scale that offers a somewhat structured clinical interview outline for clinicians. The Brown (1995) scales, mentioned above, are available for adults, and Conners (1995) developed an ADHD history form for adults to complete. Other self-report scales for adults have been developed by Nadeau (1995), Triolo (1995), Copeland (1994), and Barkley (1991). Table 2.1 provides a summary of diagnostic scales and checklists used with child, adolescent, and adult populations.

The Continuous Performance Tests (CPT)

A variety of computer-generated continuous performance tests (CPT) have been developed that utilize the presentation of visual stimuli to identify ADHD symptoms of impulsivity and inattention. These CPTs include the Test of Variables of Attention (TOVA) and the Gordon Diagnostic System (Gordon, 1986; Gordon & Metelman, 1988). One study reported that the introduction of Ritalin to a sample of ADHD adolescents significantly improved the respondents' response time and accuracy on the CPT (Klorman et al., 1991). While these tests can be interesting and stimulating for both the clinician and the test participant because of the interaction with the computer, they measure only a narrow range of responses to visual stimuli. As we have mentioned, many ADHD individuals have far more difficulty with auditory stimuli. Barkley (1994) reported that in his study of these instruments, the CPTs identified only three out of every five children previously diagnosed with ADHD. Considerable literature is available (Halperin et al., 1988; Prescott, 1993; Seidle & Joschko, 1990) discussing the relative reliability of the CPTs. There are also unanswered questions concerning the influence of gender on the comparative response rates in the CPTs (Greenberg & Waldman, 1993; Seidel & Joschko, 1991).

We are concerned that these CPTs are too often used as a "shortcut" for screening and, in some cases, confirmation of ADHD diagnoses. In our practices we often encounter ADHD individuals, usually children or adolescents, who reported having been screened by private "ADHD specialists" or commercial educational and tutoring centers using only the CPT. Many of these students' parents were told that their child did not have ADHD because the CPT was an "accurate" measure of the disorder. Other parents, whose children scored poorly on the CPT, reported that their child was "diagnosed on the spot" with ADHD. For some of these students it was later determined that they were either LD, with visual processing deficits, or a combination of ADHD and LD. These tests should *never* be utilized as a sole diagnostic indicator of ADHD. Clinicians need to be aware that their overall reliability remains questionable. We do not use CPTs in our practices and regard their results cautiously when they appear in a student's records.

THE ROLE OF MEDICAL CONSULTATION AND INTERVENTION

Because of the bioneurological and medical implications of ADHD, the nonmedical clinician must develop working relationships with physicians whose specialties are family medicine, pediatrics, and child and/or adult psychiatry. Many individuals diagnosed with ADHD—whether children, adolescents, or adults—may benefit particularly from the stimulant medications. In fact, these medications may be crucial to the processes of both the ADHD individual gaining control over her or his symptoms and utilizing the therapeutic efforts to create successes and restore self-esteem. Many diagnosed patients may already have had experience with a variety of prescribed medications with varying results, particularly if they were not prescribed or monitored by physicians experienced in working with ADHD.

The role of the physician as a consultant to the therapist is essential to the overall ADHD evaluation process, particularly in regard to the following areas:

1. Evaluating the individual's physical status and relative needs prior to prescribing medications.
2. Prescribing, monitoring, and adjusting the medications when necessary.
3. Evaluating individuals who have been prescribed stimulant medications from other medical sources but where the therapeutic levels appear ineffective.
4. Providing ongoing consultation, follow-up, and medical management.

In some cases referral to a pediatric neurologist may be necessary. This medical resource is critical; the therapist who develops a network of knowledgeable consulting physicians can provide valuable therapeutic services to his or her ADHD patients.

It is a deep relief to ADHD patients when the therapist can immediately call a physician's office to make a referral. In seeking affiliation with medical colleagues and consultants, we have found that it is equally important for the physician to value working collaboratively with other professionals and to be available to consult with the therapist and the ADHD families in treatment. A lot of clinical time can be spent working with an "unknown" physician who has to be educated and "convinced" that the clinician's evaluation and the ADHD diagnosis are proper and that the child could benefit from medication. There are certainly many pediatricians who take seriously an ADHD diagnosis and the child's and family's struggles but who simply do not have sufficient experience prescribing and overseeing the course of these medications, particularly for very young children, older adolescents, or adults. Occasionally, some of the physicians with whom we have worked closely will ask *us* if we feel the dosage is appropriate or effective for the patients.

It is important for therapists to understand the roles and responsibilities of physicians, both technically and politically. Over the years we have found that child psychiatrists, in general, appear to be the most available to other professionals and are the most willing to work medically with ADHD children and adolescents. A number of nonpsychiatric physicians, whose specialties are in family medicine, internal medicine, or pediatrics, have shared with us their hesitation to accept too many ADHD referrals from us because the stimulant medications are classified and monitored as "controlled substances." They are concerned that if they prescribe many of these controlled medications, they risk review by their state medical board or an audit of their records. A couple of the physicians with whom we have worked over the years have reported to us that they have indeed been reviewed because of their use of Ritalin with children, and that they had to produce records and other documents to support their prescriptions. Other physicians, particularly ones who have referred patients to us with positive results, will prescribe stimulants for their own patients but only after we have evaluated their ADHD patient and sent them a written statement of our diagnosis with a recommendation for the use of medication.

The issue of medication for ADHD adults raises other concerns for therapists. Many physicians and adult psychiatrists are simply not aware of the research and literature on the existence of adult ADHD. Some continue to identify ADHD as a "childhood disorder." Some internal medicine and family practice physicians are willing to medicate adults who have ADHD if the diagnosis is confirmed by a therapist. However, many of these physicians do not have enough experience to try alternative medications or to effectively "fine-tune" the dosages for some individuals. We have found that child psychiatrists as a group are the most experienced with the stimulant medications, and therefore are more effective in prescribing for ADHD adults. Unfortunately, many child psychiatrists are not willing to see patients over 18 years of age. Moreover, many adult psychiatrists tell us that they do not support medicating adults for ADHD. Thus clinicians need to search carefully for physicians who are willing and able to be helpful participants in consulting for the treatment of adult ADHD. Most psychiatrists, particularly those specializing in working with children, typically have very busy schedules, so therapists will benefit from developing a relationship with several so that any one does not feel overwhelmed by referrals.

We are fortunate to have worked with several knowledgeable and personable child and adult psychiatrists and a behavioral pediatric specialist who value the role of working with the families of ADHD patients. However, in our own community there are very few adult psychiatrists who specialize in working with adult ADHD. Based on feedback we receive at national workshops, we understand this to be a fairly widespread reality. We have developed reciprocal relationships with several of these physicians, whereby we make referrals to them for a medical evaluation and include them in consultations for evaluation and treatment of ADHD adults. In turn, these physicians refer their potential ADHD patients to us either for further clinical evaluation before medication decisions are made or for ongoing therapy. We are also fortunate to have a psychiatrist in our practice group who works with both children and adults. Often we will invite him to join us in session with the ADHD individual and her or his parents or spouse to consult about treatment planning and medical issues. This is a very effective professional relationship and has provided immediate and efficient clinical services to our ADHD families.

The Use and Effectiveness of Medications

Determining the use of medications in the treatment of ADHD is a critical part of the evaluation process and a continuing concern in overall treatment strategies and planning. Some families require considerable time during the evaluation to discuss recommendations regarding and consequences of the use of medications. Therefore, we will address the issue of medication here, in the context of evaluations, since the implications of decisions made at this time will affect all following clinical interventions.

Most experts in the field agree that medication has been, and continues to be, the "single most effective treatment for ADD" (Quinn, 1997). The beneficial effects of medication on the broad range of ADHD symptoms can often be no less than "amazing" in all three clinical populations of children, adolescents, and adults. Psychostimulants have been utilized with hyperactive children for over 50 years, and have an even longer history of use with other psychiatric disorders (Quinn, 1997; Warneke, 1990). However, therapists who work with ADHD patients encounter increasing resistance from parents about the use of stimulant medication, particularly Ritalin (methylphenidate), since it is the most widely used and has been the best known over several decades. Many families have "heard horror stories" about Ritalin from friends or neighbors or have read negative reports in the media. They report being told that it makes children behave "like zombies" or that "they could lose so much weight" their health could be jeopardized. Unfortunately, like Prozac, which is widely used for treating depression, stimulant medications have been subjected to unfair negative attacks throughout the media.

Many parents have already heard of or read stories about the potential "bad effects" of stimulant medications, their "long-term problems" or their "misuse" or their "overuse to control children." Some parents will state, in effect, "I don't want my child to turn into a zombie." In order to address these serious concerns, the nonmedical clinician working with ADHD populations *must become educated about the general pharmacology of the medications used to treat ADHD, their potential side effects, how their usage is prescribed, and the specific benefits of their use in practical behavioral terms.* It is often helpful to give families a short handout that provides an overview of the use of medications with ADHD (Miller's [1994] "Guide" is concise and readable). An effective review of general pharmacological issues in the treatment of ADHD is presented by Wilens (1998) and Wilens and Biederman (1992).

The controversy surrounding the use of stimulants in the treat- ✓ ment of ADHD has arisen due to the relatively dramatic increase in their usage over the past decade. Quinn (1997) estimated that prescriptions written for the three primary stimulant medications—Ritalin, Dexedrine, and Cylert—"have tripled from 1990 to 1994," with approximately *750,000 to 1.6 million individuals* currently taking the medications. However, Quinn (1997) also pointed out (and we agree with her observation) that this dramatic increase is not a sign of misuse but instead a product of (1) better clinical and medical detection and diagnosis and (2) the growing number of adults with ADHD now seeking treatment.

Beyond the media controversies, many parents are rightfully protective when it comes to making a decision to medicate their children, whether the stimulants are perceived as "magical cures" or "evil control mechanisms." An interesting study investigated the comparative attitudes of nonparental adults toward the use of psychotropic medications with school-age boys who had either ADHD or a seizure disorder (Summers & Caplan, 1987). The adults perceived the parents of the ADHD children as being less justified in using medications than the parents of the epileptic children. The adults also expressed concerns that the use of drugs with the ADHD children would "exacerbate the behavioral problems" more than for the epileptic children. Parents of young children, particularly preschoolers and first- and second-graders are particularly wary of medications, even though they may recognize the disruptive effects of early hyperactivity on their child's development. Clinicians need to respect these parental concerns and must address their fears with sensitivity and credibility.

Many parents have shared with us their unhappy and distasteful experiences with teachers, school counselors, pediatricians, and other therapists who tried to make them feel guilty for asking questions and hesitating to medicate their ADHD child. Some parents report having been "ordered" by preschool program directors or even teachers in the early grades of private school to get their child medicated or "don't bother to bring him back." Clearly, the motivation of such admonishments was behavioral control in the classroom, not the best interests of the children. For a therapist, teacher, or even a physician to "push" medications onto wary parents, to not take time to be a sympathetic listener before making recommendations, or to use guilt to try to convince parents of the value of medication is irresponsible. Moreover, such actions undermine parents' trust in the therapist and their sense of self-respect—both of which are vitally necessary for effective ongoing treatment.

The overall effectiveness of the stimulants for use with children is estimated by Quinn (1997) at 75–85%; in an earlier study Barkley (1990) estimated 60–80%. The range of Ritalin's effectiveness with ADHD adolescents is reported at similar levels by Wilens and Beiderman (1992) at a rate of 75%. In fact, as early as 1977 Barkley reported the benefits of Ritalin in decreasing the ADHD child's activity levels and increasing her or his ability to focus attention. The overall benefits to ADHD *children,* in both symptom reduction and improved behaviors, include (Barkley, 1990a; Wender, 1995):

1. Reduced hyperactivity and restlessness at home and in the classroom.
2. Decreased impulsivity.
3. Increased attention, concentration, and short-term memory.
4. Decreased lability.
5. Decreased frequency and level of reactivity and temper outbursts.

In a controlled study with grade school-age ADHD boys, Hinshaw and his colleagues (1989) reported that the use of Ritalin decreased physical retaliation and enhanced self-control when subjects were confronted by peer provocation. In general, Ritalin appears to be less effective in improving problematic social skills and in decreasing oppositional and aggressive behaviors (Quinn, 1997), or in improving some patterns of cognitive functioning that fall in the gray areas between ADHD and specific LD (which we will discuss later). Based on controlled studies with grade school-age ADHD boys, Cook and his colleagues (1993) reported that central auditory processing disorder symptoms, which we find are present and may affect many ADHD students' cognitive functioning in school, are so closely related to ADHD that they could be used as an effective measure of it. Cook and colleagues (1993) reported that children with central auditory processing disorders as well as ADHD symptoms responded favorably to Ritalin.

For adults, the effectiveness of stimulant medications for ADHD is estimated to be 50% by Quinn (1997) and up to 75% by Barkley (1997). Wilens and his colleagues (1995a) reviewed the use of stimulants with ADHD adults and reported that data from controlled studies were more "equivocal," ranging from 25–78%, as compared to a consistent 70% for their use with ADHD children. E. Wender's (1985, 1995) studies on ADHD *adults* reported beneficial effects from the medications that were similar to those with children:

1. Ability to sit still for longer periods and attend to present activities such as dinner or television.
2. Improved concentration.
3. Decreased distractibility.
4. Improved perseverance and completion of tasks.
5. Decreased impatience and impulsivity.
6. Decreased mood lability and boredom.

We have seen many ADHD adults who, when medicated, have regained their confidence in reading and learning and decided to return to school to complete their educations. Many had been high school dropouts. Some of these ADHD adults, now in midlife, have completed their high school diplomas and continued on to college successfully. Wender reported an ADHD adult who had read only a couple of books in his lifetime. After beginning use of a stimulant medication he "developed a passion for reading and consumed nonfiction as well as fiction at the rate of a book per week" (Wender, 1995, p. 31).

Characteristics of the Medications

Ritalin

Ritalin (methylphenidate) is the most widely (90%) prescribed of the stimulant medications (Culbert et al., 1994). It is available in 5-mg dosages and in scored 10-mg and 20-mg tablets. Ritalin-SR (slow release) is a longer acting 20-mg form. There has been some controversy regarding the latter, in that the manufacturer's data suggest that it will last for 8 hours, while most practitioners have observed a considerably shorter duration of 4 to 5 hours. Wender (1995) recommended that its duration should be observed on a "trial and error" basis.

The typical dosages of Ritalin range 15–90 mg per day. Effects of the medication are experienced within 30 to 90 minutes after the dose is taken. Wender (1995) recommended beginning with a 5-mg dose and increasing this by 5 mg every 2 to 3 days. Since the effective duration of Ritalin is fairly short (2 to 4 hours), he recommended that it be taken every 3 hours up to four times per day. He also emphasized the need to take it consistently in order to avoid what has been called a "rebound" or "roller coaster" effect. This occurs when the effective therapeutic level of the medication begins to wear off before the next dosage is administered. The symptoms of this rebound usually include increased hyperactivity, headaches, and irritability (Quinn, 1997). Wender (1995) advises his ADHD patients to use wristwatch alarms and timers to aid them in remembering when to take the medications on a consistent schedule. This may be helpful for many ADHD adults who have difficulty remembering scheduled responsibilities.

For children and adolescents, there are many recommended schedules for the use of Ritalin and other stimulants. Most will take their initial dose with, or after, breakfast. Their second dose is usually administered by the school nurse or other official before lunch at school. A third dose may be taken after the student has returned home following school. Many students and adults do not take a dose later than 5:00 P.M. because it can occasionally produce insomnia if it has not cleared their systems by bedtime. The use of the sustained- or slow-release medication can be helpful for some children and adolescents, particularly those who resist, or feel embarrassed about, going to the nurse's office at their school to receive their midday dose. However, as we pointed out, the effectiveness of the slow-release medication can subside by midday.

Children who display considerable hyperactivity may be prescribed the slow-release Ritalin and have it supplemented with 5–10 mg full-dosage tablets in the mornings and midday. Often it can be useful to combine the slow-release and rapid-acting forms to obtain maximum benefits. A variety of combinations to meet the idiosyncratic needs and situations of each individual can be created: for example, a slow-release dose in the mornings followed by a short-acting dose after lunch, or a short-acting dose in the mornings followed by a slow-release one at lunchtime. Wilens and his colleagues (1995a) reported that no studies were available on the effectiveness of the sustained-release Ritalin or Dexedrine with ADHD adults.

Dexedrine

Dexedrine (dextroamphetamine) is approximately twice as potent as Ritalin and thus the prescribed dosage is about half (E. Wender, 1995). Dexedrine is effective for 3 to 4 hours and is usually initially prescribed at 2.5 mg three to four times per day at 3 to 4 hour intervals. It can then be increased by 2.5 mg every 3 to 4 days. The average dosage per day is 15–45 mg. The longer acting Dexedrine is available in 5-, 10-, and 15-mg sizes and can produce an initial "spike" effect involving either agitation or sedation symptoms (Wender, 1995). Both Dexedrine and Ritalin have comparable effectiveness and are selected more on the basis of the physician's personal preference.

In terms of side effects, both Ritalin and Dexedrine, when taken at an excessive dosage level, can produce agitation. Dexedrine can also produce sedation or what patients describe as "fogginess" or feeling like a "zombie." Other side effects include dry mouth, loss of appetite, and weight loss (Barkley et al., 1990). This latter can be a concern for some underweight children or early adolescents and may require special management and nutritional supplements (Quinn, 1997). Some underweight children need to be watched closely so that the medications do not produce further weight loss.

Sleep disorders are sometimes reported as a problem, particularly if either medication is taken late in the day. Difficulty falling asleep or not being able to sleep through the night, as well as difficulty waking up in the mornings, are typical sleep-related complaints. However, for some "overaroused" ADHD individuals, Ritalin may actually normalize sleep patterns (Quinn, 1997). There is also a concern regarding hypertension (E. Wender, 1995). The physician typically examines a patient's medical history with particular concern for cardiac and kidney disorders and any other medical concerns that might be a contraindication for using stimulants.

Neither of these medications has been associated with allergic reactions, and tolerance to either is rare; most patients "experience no decrease in efficacy even after years of use" (Wender, 1995, p. 171). However, Quinn (1997) reported that tolerance to a particular stimulant may occur after several years, which then requires substituting another stimulant.

Overall, Barkley and his colleagues (1990) reported that, in a controlled study of 83 ADHD children taking Ritalin, only three of the children experienced side effects severe enough to warrant discontinuation of the medication. In this study the parents reported increased side effects of appetite loss, insomnia, headaches, and stomachaches.

Wilens and associates (1995a) noted that studies that used stimulant medications with ADHD adults have reported only "mild" side effects, the most common being "insomnia, edginess, diminished appetite, weight loss, dysphoria, and headaches." However, they also noted that "the long-term adverse effects and sustained efficacy of the stimulants in adults with ADHD remain unstudied" (p. 273).

Cylert

Cylert (pemoline) is another stimulant medication used fairly widely, until recently, in the treatment of ADHD. Its effectiveness is somewhat less (77%) than that of Dexedrine (96%) and it can take up to 8 weeks to achieve full potency, as compared to 2 weeks for Dexedrine (Quinn, 1997). However, more recent studies have suggested that at higher dosages the medication can be effective more quickly (Pelham et al., 1995; Quinn, 1997). E. Wender (1995) reported that Cylert was effective in a smaller proportion of ADHD patients and that some responded to it better than to the other stimulants. Similarly, Wilens and colleagues' (1995a) review of stimulant medications with ADHD adults reported that the effectiveness of Cylert was comparable to that of Ritalin.

Cylert is prescribed in a dosage range of 18.75–150 mg per day. Potential side effects with Cylert include anorexia, abdominal discomfort, headaches, and insomnia. Wender (1995) noted that this medication must be monitored with laboratory screening since cases of elevated liver enzymes, hepatitis, jaundice, and aplastic anemia have been reported in association with it. In fact, *a recent bulletin from the pharmaceutical company warned of specific concerns regarding potential liver problems.*

Cylert is classified as a Schedule IV drug, which means it is less likely to be abused than Ritalin and Dexedrine, which are classified as Schedule II drugs. There have been increasing reports regarding abuse of Ritalin and Dexedrine. In most cases these medications need to be ingested at high doses, either intravenously or "snorted," to produce euphoric effects. One clinical report identified the case of an adolescent who had accumulated Ritalin for several days and "snorted" 100 mg to produce a "high" (Jaffe, 1991). Clinicians need to be aware of the ADHD patient's history of substance abuse or risk of such (Wender, 1995).

Adderall

Adderall is a new stimulant medication that is a derivative of amphetamines, but its use has not yet been reported in the literature. It is available in 5-, 10-, 20-, and 30-mg scored tablets and can be prescribed at a dosage up to 40 mg per day. Its side effects are similar to those with Ritalin or Dexedrine.

Antidepressants

Antidepressants have been reported as effective with some ADHD patients; however, extensive research regarding their usage is still lacking. Prozac (fluoxetine) has been reported to have moderate benefits with few side effects in some clinical experiences with ADHD children and adolescents (Wilens et al., 1995a; Wilens, 1998). Wender (1995) reported that he found Prozac to be ineffective with ADHD patients, though he admitted his experience with it was limited. Wellbutrin (bupropion) has been reported as helpful for ADHD children (Casat et al., 1987; Simeon et al., 1986) as well as adults (Wender & Reimherr, 1990). Tofranil (imipramine) is also prescribed for ADHD.

These medications are most effective when a comorbid depression is present (Quinn, 1997). Wender (1995) has observed that Wellbutrin is often more effective for ADHD symptoms where depression is present and it is combined with a stimulant. Wilens and associates (1995) noted that most reports on the use of antidepressants with ADHD adults are largely anecdotal and that effective, controlled studies are still needed.

Catapres (clonidine) and Tenex (guanfacine) are also used with ADHD, particularly with those children who display greater hyperactivity and anxiety, as well as those with a concurrent tic disorder (Quinn, 1997).

Clinical Issues in the Use of Medications

We support the therapeutic use of stimulants and/or other medications with ADHD patients, whether children, adolescents, or adults, whenever we feel that the medications will effectively reduce symptoms and help the individuals gain control over their life experiences. As we have discussed, parents and ADHD individuals have a right to have their questions answered and their fears addressed so that they can make an informed decision about beginning the use of a medication. We try to provide as much up-to-date information about these medications as possible to the families with whom we work.

We also make it clear to families that none of these medications offers a "cure" for ADHD. We stress that medications will temporarily help the individual function more effectively in her or his everyday life. Miller (1994) used the analogy of medications as "supportive" treatment, much like insulin is for diabetes or eyeglasses are for vision problems. We emphasize that medication alone will not solve all of the individual's problems and explain the value and the role of ongoing therapy for both the ADHD individual and her or his family.

We have found that, in addition to explaining the medical issues, it is helpful to discuss with parents the possible positive effects of the medication on an ADHD child's self-esteem. Most parents of ADHD children are quite aware of how the constant barrage of criticism and negative feedback they receive at home and school erodes their self-confidence and personal resources. We explain to the parents that this dramatic and chronic pattern of negative feedback can be interrupted, often within days, by the use of medication, and that ongoing treatment with the family can begin to repair prior damage to their child's self-esteem.

Based on our respective 20-plus years of working with ADHD children, we believe strongly that the use of stimulant medications can rapidly facilitate the individual's functioning and diffuse many symptoms almost immediately. These beneficial effects enhance the process of therapy, whether the focus is on the stabilization of the individual and family; on the individual's response to accommodations at school, home, or work; or on self-esteem issues. We also know from our clinical experiences that often the most structured and thoughtful therapeutic plan, including the enlistment of school cooperation and accommodations, may fail dramatically without the use of medication.

Nevertheless, many parents, motivated either by misinformation or simply concern about medicating their child, will ask us, "Can't we try other methods before we have to use medicine?" A few parents have said to us, "We would rather bring our child to see you three or four times a week than put her [him] on pills everyday." The therapist needs to be sensitive to these parental concerns. In cases where we feel strongly that stimulant medication is indicated for treatment success but the parents remain unconvinced, and we have used all of our psychoeducational resources (including sometimes a brief consultation with a physician), we will reluctantly develop an alternative treatment plan.

In one such case the single mother of an extremely hyperactive first-grade boy sought our consultation because the teacher and school principal felt that her son was often unmanageable in class and they had received complaints from the parents of other children that he was "rough and intimidating." The boy's father had been killed in an industrial accident several years earlier and the mother had become excessively overprotective of her only child. The diagnosis of ADHD, hyperactive–impulsive type, was made, but the mother refused the recommendation of stimulant medication. She said, "He is so young and vulnerable. How can I make him take this medicine?" We helped her develop an alternative treatment plan, which called for her to enforce more structured behavioral controls at home. We consulted with the teacher and gave her some suggestions for helping focus and maintain the child's attention in class. We also encouraged the mother to begin to leave her child with a babysitter so that she could occasionally go out with friends and develop a social life.

The mother's efforts to enforce behavioral management strategies at home were halfhearted due to her habitual overprotectiveness. The teacher followed through on our suggestions quite effectively, but the mother became critical of the teacher for "being unsupportive" and trying to "overcontrol" her son. The mother had responded to the suggestion to pursue some social activities, but after three attempts she was quite discouraged. Each of the three babysitters she had employed had refused to return again to babysit her son. They all complained that he was "too hyper" and "unmanageable." This did get her attention, and she asked us what to do. We had recently heard from the teacher that she was not having much success with the boy in the classroom and that she was also frustrated by the mother's continued criticism of her efforts.

We suggested to the mother that she take an afternoon off from work and sit quietly in the back of her son's classroom for 2 hours as a silent observer. Reluctantly, she agreed. We made a list for the mother of the kinds of things she could look for in observing her son. (We have found this to be a helpful intervention for many parents, though we have learned that we need to challenge them to remain focused on their child rather than evaluating the teacher's actions.) This list of items included comparing her son's level of activity with those of his classmates, his ability to remain in his seat for specific periods of time, his degree of restlessness or talkativeness, and the amount of time he spent listening to the teacher as compared to fidgeting with items on his desk or rocking in his chair. We even suggested that she use her watch to time her son's attention span while he was either completing work at his desk or while the teacher was speaking.

This experience served as a dramatic turning point for the mother: she finally comprehended the severity of her son's disruptiveness and his inability to stay focused and on task in the classroom. When she met with us later she said, "I kept looking down at my watch, like you suggested, but he never settled down for more than a minute or two. That's just like he is at home. Do you really think the medication would help him?" The child was placed on Ritalin and manifested such clearly effective results the next day at school that the teacher called us that afternoon to tell us that the medication was "like magic." Most of the ensuing therapy was focused on teaching the mother better child management skills—which, of course, were more effective now that her child was successfully medicated—and helping her process the grief of the loss of her husband so that she could begin to gain some independence from her child and go on with her life as an adult.

In the following chapter we will examine more closely the multiple roles in which the therapist can function in order to enhance the treatment of ADHD, and the usefulness of developing an interdisciplinary network of consultants.

APPENDIX 2.1. SAMPLE REFERRAL LETTER FOR PSYCHOEDUCATIONAL TESTING

Dear Dr. Smith:

I am referring my patient, Mark Jones, to you for testing to support the potential diagnosis of ADHD. Mark is an 8-year-old student in the third grade at River Bend Elementary School. According to both his teacher's and parents' reports he displays many symptoms consistent with ADHD: short attention span, distractibility, poor short-term memory, restlessness in the classroom, occasional confrontations with other students, excessive talkativeness, and he is below grade level in reading and math. I am attaching a copy of the *ACTerS* screening profile that was completed by his teacher. His parents are in a disagreement about the potential of ADHD and are also considering a separation. There is the possibility that the father may also have ADHD.

There were also reports that Mark Jones may have been periodically depressed and as recently as 3 weeks ago sat at the teacher's desk crying for no apparent reason. In addition to the WISC-III and the WJ-R, I would suggest that you administer a brief depression scale. I will be working with him in individual and family therapy. He is not medicated at this time, though we are considering a trial on stimulants pending the support of the diagnosis by your evaluation.

Please feel free to give me a call if I can give you additional information. A release signed by his mother is also attached.

Sincerely,

Craig A. Everett, PhD

3

Interdisciplinary Issues and Multiple Responsibilities of the Therapist

To effectively evaluate ADHD and to implement realistic treatment strategies, the therapist invariably becomes involved in processing a broad range of clinical information and developing multiple levels of interventions. In contrast to the initial treatment of patients with other psychiatric disorders, the therapist treating an ADHD patient will need not only extensive data regarding the ADHD individual's and family's history but also collaborative information from parents, teachers, and school counselors if the patient is a child or adolescent, and from spouses and family-of-origin members if the patient is an adult. The specific treatment strategies we recommend involve working with broader and more complex clinical dynamics and interactional patterns than one encounters in more traditional individual psychotherapy. When treating ADHD, the therapist may need to define a clinical role and a working relationship with multiple family members, extended family subsystems, and other community professionals. The clinician may find that she or he needs to conduct therapy sessions with up to five or six family members at a time in order, for example, to effectively challenge the family's problematic dynamics that have been focused on an ADHD child. The clinician will also need to define her or his therapeutic role carefully due to the complex assessment and treatment needs of ADHD patients and their families. Even the most experienced family therapist will not be able to meet all these various responsibilities. We have learned that the clinician's role will be enhanced by consulting and collaborating with other professionals, such as physicians, psychometrists, school personnel, and even attorneys.

We thought that it would be helpful to provide an overview of the various resources we have integrated into our clinical practices to focus and enhance our work with ADHD patients. We want to do this in a practical way to inform the therapist regarding both clinical approaches and practice management issues. Even though we specialize in working with children, families, and spouses, we found that we needed to develop more astuteness in eliciting comprehensive histories and in developing specific diagnostic procedures that tracked the ADHD symptoms across childhood experiences and even into adulthood. We also learned the importance of psychoeducational evaluations and how to use testing data for both diagnostic and therapeutic purposes.

Another resource that we cultivated was the provision of psycho-educational information to ADHD individuals and their families. We find the provision of specific information about ADHD, as well as information about the broader areas of parenting, communication, and marital and family interaction, indispensable. We believe that teaching ADHD families how found that learning to integrate basic psychoeducational information about parent–child interactions, family dynamics, and the cluster of ADHD symptoms can be immensely helpful because it gives them a clearer sense of how the symptoms are affecting their child's ability to learn and succeed in school, as well as how they have a continuing impact on their home and family environment. We have learned that many families respond well to basic information about managing their daily life experiences more effectively or improving their parenting and communication skills. Of course, some cases will also require more complex clinical interventions.

It is highly advisable, even crucial, for therapists working with ADHD patients to develop effective interdisciplinary relationships. In our work with ADHD families, the process of ongoing collaboration and consultation with other professionals has become central to our clinical effectiveness.

Over the years of our professional work, we have also been involved in the preparation of clinical evaluations in child custody disputes for attorneys and the courts. Early in our careers we served as directors of a court-sponsored family and child advocacy program where we developed a family-focused team approach to working with custody evaluations (Everett & Volgy, 1983). We were familiar with the roles of a clinician in legal and court settings, and we found this familiarity useful in preparing us to work with difficult ADHD family situations that involved not only divorce factors but other legal complications such as delinquency, probation, and criminal charges against patients.

Perhaps the role that we function in most extensively in our work with ADHD families is that of advocacy. Certainly all therapists perform limited services as advocates for their clients, be they children, adults, or families. However, in most clinical situations, particularly marital and family contexts, an advocacy role must be tempered so that the therapist is free to work with both the system as a whole and each of its members. To become aligned with any one family member can severely limit the therapist's effectiveness with the entire family, unless the temporary alliance is related to a clearly developed intervention. Many family therapists may become advocates for the entire family, not just the individuals whom they are treating. We have found that advocacy is a central part of the therapist's ongoing clinical role with ADHD families. For example, when working with ADHD children and adolescents, the therapist may be called upon to become an advocate in school or court settings. In working with ADHD adults, the therapist may become an advocate in the work setting to help them secure accommodations that adhere to federal disability guidelines, within their marriages and families, and occasionally in the courts.

The therapist's role in effectively treating ADHD can become complex and often quite time-consuming. The type of clinical structures that therapists develop and their definitions of specific roles can clarify their interventions and maximize their effectiveness. We encourage therapists to examine the variety of roles that we will discuss here and determine for themselves the specific clinical areas where they can become most effective, based on their training, orientation, and even personality styles. The other roles that we recommend for effective treatment with ADHD families can be developed by therapists through consultation and collaborative relationships.

In this chapter we will discuss the clinical resources that are crucial ingredients for effective practice with ADHD patients, including the following:

1. Developing an interdisciplinary network.
2. Consulting with educational specialists.
3. Consulting with attorneys.
4. Advocacy in school and work settings.
5. Advocacy with other professionals.
6. Advocacy regarding legal issues.
7. A psychoeducational role.

THE IMPORTANCE OF DEVELOPING AN INTERDISCIPLINARY NETWORK

Our experience with ADHD families has taught us that a therapist working alone is much less effective clinically in responding to the complex therapeutic needs of ADHD individuals and their families compared to the therapist who uses a team or network of consulting specialists. Few of us have been trained to handle a range of expertise that includes such specializations as psychoeducational testing, psychopharmacology, educational consultation, and the legal interpretation of federal disabilities guidelines. Even with training in all of these clinical specialties, few therapists in either independent or agency practices could, by themselves, meet the variety of needs of these ADHD families.

Many experienced therapists do not consult or collaborate with other professionals except when faced with an emergency or a highly problematic situation. This weakness is typically due to the time and structural requirements of independent practice. Over the years we have tried to focus our roles more realistically in terms of what we believe we can do best, and then supplement the remaining areas via a network of effective professional consultants with whom we can collaborate for additional resources. We strongly believe that the most effective therapeutic outcomes are achieved when multiple professionals are involved in the diagnosis, educational planning, and ongoing treatment of ADHD individuals.

Experience and comfort with professional collaboration are important. Early in our work in the ADHD field, we became involved with many families who were referred to us due to a child's school problems. However, in many of these cases other therapists were involved in treating the child's behavioral problems or the parental and marital problems. In some of these cases psychiatrists were also involved, often working with one of the other therapists in treating and medicating one of the parents for some other emotional disorder, or medicating the child for a comorbid condition. Because of the multiple levels of clinical problems in ADHD families, many families will have been in therapy previously or will be currently involved with other therapists for a variety of clinical reasons, but not necessarily for diagnosed ADHD. The professionals that we believe are essential for collaboration in assessing and treating ADHD include (1) a psychometrist, (2) a physician, (3) an educational consultant, (4) a career specialist, and (5) an attorney.

We receive many referrals to work with a child previously diagnosed with ADHD. Often we find that teachers, a school counselor, a school psychologist, a principal, a pediatrician, and a psychiatrist are already involved in the case and already offering a broad range of clinical advice to the family. But in the majority of these cases no clear clinical or educational plan incorporating the broader systemic needs and resources of the family has been developed. If there is a focused treatment plan, it generally does not take into consideration such dynamics as parental and sibling roles in relation to the ADHD child or underlying marital dynamics. In fact, in many of these cases it is not uncommon for the various professionals, clinical as well as educational, to be at odds with one another's recommendations. Parents often tell us that they feel bewildered and overwhelmed by the volume of conflicting advice they receive from these differing professionals. Some educational specialists working with ADHD children resent or are intimidated by what they perceive as intrusiveness by clinical professionals, just as some clinicians who are privately treating a child's ADHD may ignore or outrightly devalue the professional resources of the educational specialists.

As we worked with these types of entangled cases, we would find ourselves, at times, being pulled into alliances with competing professionals. For example, a school psychologist or principal might challenge us to justify the development of specific educational accommodations for an ADHD student, even though they had been previously requested by a parent. Or a teacher might try to talk us into supporting her or his recommendation for medicating the ADHD child, even though the parents had expressed great reluctance to use medications. Or we were asked by parents to intervene on the child's behalf with their pediatrician to convince her or him either to consider medicating their ADHD child or to reevaluate the apparent ineffectiveness of the child's present medication.

We have often found ourselves, somewhat naively at first, assuming an advocacy role for the ADHD child or adolescent in the midst of this professional confusion and conflict. This alliance would often lead to stress in our relationship with the parents. Gradually, however, we learned that it was much more effective therapeutically to develop advocacy roles for the family system as a whole, not just for the ADHD individual.

As we learned to clarify a more effective clinical role with ADHD families, we found that we could be instrumental in helping to develop and coordinate resources for a more complete ADHD evaluation and treatment process for families. Having already experienced the many personal and professional political traps that arise when working with other clinicians, physicians, and educators, we could easily identify with the feelings of bewilderment and helplessness that many ADHD families expressed. We also became quite critical of the harm often done to ADHD students when their families are left on their own to deal with the competing agendas of educators and therapists. For example:

A therapist tells parents that their child should be tested, while the educators tell the parents testing is unnecessary.

Teachers pressure parents to have their hyperactive child medicated, while their pediatrician tells them that their child is too young to be medicated.

A therapist tells parents that their child is diagnosed as having a conduct disorder and little can be done to improve her or his behaviors, while at the same time the teachers are telling the parents that their child is in danger of failing and they had better do something.

These and other frustrating experiences taught us that ADHD families not only need effective evaluation and treatment services, but also access to professionals who could coordinate these services. This led us to develop a variety of interdisciplinary relationships with professionals who were well trained in their own specialities and knowledgeable about the complex aspects of ADHD, and upon whom we could easily call for either consultation or collaboration. With our ADHD families, we often refer to these interdisciplinary relationships as our "ADHD team," even though there are no formally defined relationships and everyone practices in separate locations. For ADHD families referred to us, we assume the role of coordinating and requesting services, as necessary, from members of this team. Many of these colleagues refer their own ADHD patients to us for specific services as well. Certainly, we recognize that many therapists may not wish to develop their own team approach, as we have; the alternative approach is to learn to recognize the variety of services that can benefit an ADHD family and to make appropriate referrals when necessary.

With regard to treatment issues, most of the clinical literature still focuses predominantly on the central role of cognitive or behavioral therapy for ADHD patients and the supplemental role of stimulant medications. However, there is a growing recognition of the value of a team approach in working with ADHD patients. For example, Quinn (1997) indicated that effective "multimodal" programs would include educational, psychological, social, and medical aspects of treatment, as well as offering family support, case management, and advocacy. Her statement that "whether one is treating children or adults with AD(H)D, it is particularly important to keep in mind that successful treatment should also include significant others and family members" (p. 159) certainly helps to broaden the fields's definition of treatment.

CONSULTING WITH EDUCATIONAL SPECIALISTS

As we began to take a more active advocacy role with many ADHD patients, both in the school and in work settings, it became clear that we needed to limit and focus our clinical time and resources to those areas in which we felt that we could be most effective. While both of us have taught at the graduate level in university settings, neither of us has worked in primary or secondary education. However, in addition to evaluations and accommodations, we soon found ourselves dealing with everyday issues of classroom management and structure, homework planning, and test preparations. While we could often offer helpful advice to students, parents, and even teachers regarding these issues, we did not feel that we were the best resource, nor that offering such advice was the best use of our clinical time. Therefore, some years ago we began to identify resources to help us in the role we described as "educational consultants" or learning specialists.

The need here was not simply for tutors to help ADHD students with reading or math, particularly since many school districts offer those services, but to provide broader and more practical resources at a "meta" level that would address issues of *how to study, how to take notes in class, how to keep track of homework, how to prepare for special projects, and how to prepare for examinations.* We found that individuals who had been teachers and had varying degrees of training in special education could best fill this role. Some had been educators who were no longer teaching because they did not wish to work full time but were eager to work with ADHD students a few hours a week. Special education training provides such individuals with both practical and empathic skills, beyond classroom teaching, to aid students struggling with learning problems. We have also worked, very successfully, with a Ph.D. student in education who served both a consulting role and an in-school advocacy role. She went on to complete her dissertation on working with ADHD in the classroom.

One of the most helpful consultants we have worked with, particularly with ADHD adolescents, is a young man who has his bachelor's degree in education and teaches in a local high school. He himself had dropped out of high school before he was diagnosed with ADHD. With the help of stimulant medication, he successfully completed his college degree in education. He is in his mid-20s and can talk openly about his own personal struggles in school, including the "excuses" he used to avoid work, and is helpful in discussing the value of stimulant medications as well as offering his observations and practical suggestions to ADHD children, ADHD adolescents, and their parents.

In making a referral to an educational consultant, we typically identify for the parents the exact areas of academic need for their daughter or son: for example, the ADHD student who has trouble keeping track of his assignments, either losing them or forgetting to turn them in on time; or the student who consistently procrastinates and leaves preparation for a big project or examination until the night before. A student who has struggled with algebra and simply avoids doing the homework can benefit from practical suggestions about how to study and how best to organize her time. We explain that they, as a family, whether their ADHD child is in grade school or high school, could benefit from practical consultation "to help your daughter [son] learn effective ways of studying and keeping up with her [his] work." Most parents are eager for this type of assistance because they have often tried to play this role themselves, usually with exasperation and frustration as the outcome. The therapist's referral to someone who can offer these specific skills can save parents months of often futile searching through other resources.

In complicated ADHD cases or where there appears to have been little progress, we will often review the situation in person with our educational consultants to elicit their observations, and we occasionally invite them to attend a joint meeting with the ADHD student, the parents, and ourselves. After we have worked with consultants for a period of time, and they have become acquainted with our concerns and approach, our consultants will often contact us to identify specific issues or patterns they have observed while working with a student. Occasionally they will tell us that they are having difficulty working with the parents or that the parents' marital conflicts and arguments appear to be sabotaging the student's efforts. Sometimes we ask these consultants to attend a school review or staffing meeting for the student with us, where they can play a helpful advocacy role with other teachers. The work of the educational consultant typically occurs concurrently with the therapy process, but it may also extend beyond the completion of therapy as new educational issues arise at advanced grade levels.

We also explain the work of the educational consultants to the student's parents. (In Chapter 5 we will discuss how many parents of ADHD children experience great frustration because they not only push their children to do better in school but they often take on a quasi-tutoring role with their children.) When young grade school students need help, the educational consultant works more with the parents on techniques of focusing and structuring the child's learning experiences at home. The consultant may also work with the teacher on alternative assignments and homework planning. For students in middle and high school, the consultant often works with the student and parents together. The goal here is to help the student at this age gain some successes independently and help the parents develop a more constructive role than that of "enforcer" or "nagging" parents.

We have recently begun working with a career consultant as another resource in our referral network. We are finding that this professional can be helpful to high school students as well as adults who are having difficulty focusing their career interests and preferences. Career preference testing is also available.

CONSULTING WITH ATTORNEYS

It may seem surprising that we would introduce the topic of working with attorneys and legal issues in relations to the treatment of ADHD. The relevancy becomes obvious once it is known that ADHD is recognized as a disability under federal laws with regard to both limitations and discrimination in the contexts of education and employment. As such, ADHD, along with other disabilities, is regulated by three major federal laws: the Rehabilitation Act of 1973 (RA), Section 504; the Individuals with Disabilities Education Act of 1990 (IDEA); and the Americans with Disabilities Act of 1990 (ADA).

The IDEA defines special education and services for children with disabilities. The provision of the RA and ADA termed *Section 504* identifies educational issues of which therapists need to be aware. Section 504 states that students with disabilities are entitled to *academic accommodations* and other services to enhance their learning experiences in educational settings. This "504 provision," as it is called in schools, qualifies students with general learning disabilities for services. A memorandum, issued in 1991 by the U.S. Department of Education, specified clearly the conditions under which ADHD students may be eligible for special education services under the 504 and IDEA standards. To qualify, it must be demonstrated that the ADHD student's educational experience is impaired by either physical or mental factors (Davila, Williams, & MacDonald, 1991).

The laws also address the rights of ADHD students in areas such as suspension from school and confidentiality, and define the accommodations for taking the SAT or ACT examinations. They also specify similar rights for the provision of accommodations to postsecondary ADHD students in graduate and professional schools, as well as the rights of professionals who undertake licensing examinations. Beyond educational settings, these laws also cover ADHD adults in most work settings, though certain work situations and occupations may be exempted, for example, small companies with fewer than 15 employees and occupations involving heavy machinery where the use of medication is prohibited. Obviously, ADHD adults may also benefit from legal consultation with regard to their rights in the workplace.

These federal laws are certainly recognized by school districts throughout the country. However, school districts have policies with varying interpretations of their responsibilities in both conducting evaluations and in the provision of services, specifically to ADHD students. Some school districts may have clear policies congruent with the federal guidelines, yet parents in that district may be confronted by an administrator or school psychologist whose interpretation of the student's need for an evaluation or even the range of services available may be quite restrictive. Unfortunately, sometimes it is quite difficult to gain the cooperation of school personnel in providing special services or even accommodations for their children. There are many school personnel, from school board members to teachers and counselors, who still tell parents that ADHD is just a "fad" and if their child "would just work harder he [she] would do fine."

When one of the authors (SVE) attended a 504 meeting (the designation from the Section 504 guidelines that defines the meeting of teachers, school personnel, and parents to plan accommodations for an ADHD student) at an elementary school, the principal came to the meeting with a file of magazine and newspaper articles debunking ADHD as a disability and the use of medications in its treatment. In another 504 meeting regarding a fifth-grader who had been tested and clearly diagnosed with ADHD, the principal and the special education coordinator were reluctant to provide the specific "accommodations" that we had recommended. The mother had written a letter to the school district, complaining about the lack of cooperation she was receiving from the school's staff and indicating that one of the authors (CAE) would attend the meeting. When the meeting convened, we were surprised to find that, in addition to the teacher, principal, and special education coordinator, the district superintendent and the district school psychologist were present and armed with a video camera to tape the meeting.

Often the therapist has enough influence to encourage or challenge the school personnel to develop accommodations for an ADHD student. However, when that effort is not sufficient, the family may need to employ an attorney to become an advocate for their child in gaining appropriate services. Fortunately, this need does not arise often. By now, some readers may feel that we are being too critical of schools' handling of ADHD. We certainly recognize that policies and resources range widely from state to state and district to district. But anyone working with ADHD students will hear, almost immediately, from parents about their struggles and conflicts on behalf of their child with the schools. They will typically relate in some detail their frustrations in trying to get school personnel to take seriously their child's academic difficulties, or to evaluate their child, or to provide their child with accommodations. Families who have moved frequently can often recite a continuing pattern of frustrations with the schools from state to state. For many parents these are like war stories and they may already see themselves in an adversarial role with the schools before they are referred for evaluation or therapy.

For the therapist working with ADHD patients, a responsive and knowledgeable attorney can be a valued asset in this network of professionals. We have worked with several attorneys in our community who have educated themselves about the various disability acts, even though their specialties were in other areas of law. A couple of these attorneys have children who had been diagnosed with ADHD and they were often glad to help other parents. At their annual meetings the CHADD organization (Children and Adults with Attention Deficit Disorders; see Appendix 6.1 in Chapter 6 on pages 194–195), often provides workshops for attorneys working in this area.

Typically the attorney is enlisted to write a letter to the president of a school board or to the school district's superintendent. The letter simply restates the student's diagnosis, how it was reached, and the fact that ADHD is covered under the various federal disability guidelines. In most cases, the superintendent then instructs school personnel to work with the parents and therapist to develop appropriate accommodations. In one of our cases we were disappointed because school personnel postponed a recommended evaluation of a student until the following school year because, they claimed, they did not have time to do the evaluation before the closing of school for the summer. When the superintendent received a letter from the parents' attorney, drafted at our request, the special education coordinator and the school psychologist were required to evaluate the student immediately. In another case the attorney's letter prompted a responsive school board to review the entire range of policies regarding their handling of both educational and physical disabilities. A midlevel administrator who challenged the board's proposed changes in these policies was reassigned.

Many ADHD students who are asked to take lengthy and time-limited multiple choice examinations achieve poor scores. These results are not indicative of these students' overall knowledge and achievement in high school, nor of their potential ability for college-level work. Due to the federal disabilities guidelines, the American College Test Board, which administers a number of qualifying national examinations for college entrance, including the ACT and the SAT, allows students with certain disabilities to take their tests under specially approved conditions. ADHD is a recognized disability and, when approved, ADHD high school students can take the test in a separate room and with extended time periods.

Several years ago one of the authors was working with an ADHD high school senior who, after evaluation and going on medication, had improved his grades dramatically over the first semester. The author had mentioned to the parents that if the student wanted to take the SAT the next semester, he should check into having it approved to take under these special conditions. The parents spent hours trying to convince the school counselor and the vice-principal that this was an appropriate request. The school counselor, who was an adviser for seniors planning to go to college, met with the ADHD senior and tried to "shame" him into abandoning his request: "You don't want to be put in a room by yourself to take this test. What will your friends think? If you just organize your thoughts, you can do fine taking the test with everyone else." Finally, we referred the parents to one of our legal consultants, who wrote a letter to the school board president. The necessary paper work from the school was in the mail within a week, the student took the SAT with additional time provided, and his scores were much higher than any of the school personnel had expected. He is a sophomore in college this year.

Many experienced therapists know attorneys in their community whom they can approach about working with families in this context as needed. If not, therapists might choose to become involved with their local CHADD chapter, where there may be a parent involved who is, or would know, a sympathetic attorney. In communities where there are universities with law schools, there are often special programs and offices that provide legal consultation (though not necessarily representation) to the public. Often these fall under the general title of "Law and Public Policy." The legal staff of these programs can provide useful services to the families of ADHD students.

Concerning ADHD adults, the relevancy of the federal disability acts for ADHD is not as well known by employers. However, as it does for students, the ADA protects adults from discrimination on their job due to their disability and also provides for accommodations. We suspect that there are many ADHD adults, both diagnosed and undiagnosed, who could benefit from special accommodations to enhance their work performances and perhaps increase their career longevity. Unfortunately, most of these adults are simply not aware of their rights. As therapists we often take the role of mediating with an employer by educating her or him regarding our patient's disability.

Framing the interaction as educational rather than confrontational is often quite successful, and many employers are willing to make reasonable accommodations for their employees. However, in some job contexts employers are simply not aware of their responsibilities with regard to disabilities or do not feel that they need to apply the disabilities acts to employees with "emotional/psychiatric" problems. Others may not be willing to make accommodations for a single employee. These are situations where a consultation with an attorney is important; again, most situations can be resolved by a clear and firm letter.

THE ROLE OF ADVOCACY

We have discussed how clinicians working with ADHD patients often need to assume multifaceted roles. One of the most challenging and helpful roles we perform is that of advocate for the ADHD student or employee. This concept of *advocacy* by a therapist may evoke somewhat confusing images. Most therapists are trained to be as neutral as possible. However, in reality, most therapists who work for any length of time with a patient, be it a child or an adult, will develop a sense of support and often protectiveness for that client. As noted, for therapists working with families and marriages, the issue of neutrality is often critical. The interactive dynamics of members in a family system often function to pull a therapist into taking sides or aligning with a certain member or faction of the family. If this happens without clear therapeutic intent, the clinician's ability to objectively manage the therapeutic process can be seriously jeopardized. However, because of the disabling aspects of ADHD that occur in the family, school, work, and community settings, the therapist is often in a position to play an effective role beyond the traditional clinical process in the office. Taking on an advocacy role may be a foreign notion for many clinicians who intentionally avoid involvement in issues external to the therapy setting. Many therapists are not comfortable working outside their familiar office environments. Other therapists may simply have never considered the idea of taking a broader role that would include advocacy for their ADHD patients in the school or work setting. For those who are comfortable considering adding this potential role as a resource, we will offer the following exploration of the advocacy role in a variety of settings.

Advocacy in School and Work Settings

Often recommendations from a therapist regarding an ADHD student or employee carry considerable weight in securing constructive changes and accommodations in either school or work settings. For example, when parents have been unsuccessful in gaining official consent for an educational evaluation of their son or daughter, the therapist can write a memorandum (see Appendix 3.1) to the school's officials confirming the ADHD diagnosis, explaining how it was reached, and recommending a range of potential accommodations. For another example, the therapist may be asked, by either parents or school personnel, to attend a 504 meeting (described above) to assist in developing specific accommodation plans (see appendices 3.2 and 3.3). (We will illustrate this role more specifically in Chapters 7 and 8.) Or, for ADHD adults, the therapist can write a brief letter explaining the disabling aspects of ADHD in relation to the patient's work setting and/or responsibilities, and may also attend a meeting between the ADHD employee and her or his manager(s) or supervisor. (We will illustrate this role further in Chapter 8.)

The therapist has a unique role as an ADHD educator who can help both teachers and employers better understand exactly how the disorder affects the individual and impedes her or his scholastic or work performance. Often this role involves clarifying the diagnosis and explaining the biological aspects of the disorder. Even teachers are often surprised to learn about recent research that shows growing evidence for the neurobiological basis of the disorder. Particularly in regard to employers, the therapist can offer an overview of how ADHD fits into the context of federal disability guidelines. It is our experience that this educational approach is successful in securing accommodations in 80–90% of these situations.

The other 10–20% of the time, the therapist will encounter disinterested or unsympathetic school personnel or employers. In these circumstances the therapist needs to be patient but clear and firm in explaining the patient's resources and needs. If nothing productive occurs in these initial meetings, the therapist must be prepared to move the ADHD issue to another hierarchical level. In the schools, this usually means the superintendent, and in the workplace, the owner or senior manager of a company. When the advocacy issues are discussed at these levels, the therapist must be prepared to accept a potentially more adversarial role. If this next level of meetings does not prompt constructive results, then the therapist should refer the patient to an attorney for consultation (discussed earlier).

The therapist who advocates for a single client can open doors in school and work settings for other students or employees with ADHD. On a number of occasions, particularly in school settings, after attending a 504 conference, a principal or teacher has asked us to provide an in-service training program on ADHD for the entire faculty. We have found that teachers and school counselors are quite eager to hear our perspective on ADHD. In fact, during these in-service presentations invariably a few teachers approach us to tell us that they have similar students in their classes whom they have wondered about and to express relief that now they may be better able to help them.

Advocacy with Other Professionals

Often other professionals are involved with the families of the ADHD patients we treat. For example, many families have a family pediatrician, who knows the ADHD child, other children in the family, and at least the primary caregiving parent. If medication is indicated for their ADHD child, parents might naturally prefer to work with that pediatrician. Thus the therapist making the diagnosis will need to contact the pediatrician, explain the evaluation and the diagnosis, and make a recommendation that the child be evaluated for stimulant medication. For pediatricians (or other primary care providers) who are not familiar with our work, we write out our recommendation in a brief memorandum, and then we follow up this written communication with a telephone call. Many pediatricians are knowledgeable about ADHD and treat it routinely, but even the well informed will appreciate the diagnostic support of a therapist's evaluation and recommendations.

However, this advocacy and consulting role can become more difficult if the family, either by choice or by requirement of their managed health care group, must see a primary care physician whose speciality is internal or family medicine. Here again the therapist may have to play an educational role not only in explaining the diagnosis but also assuring the physician that stimulant medication is indicated. Since many of these physicians do not prescribe these medications as frequently as pediatricians or psychiatrists, they may be reluctant to do so. The therapist's advocacy role in these cases must be clear and firm: "In my experience, ADHD individuals with these symptoms typically respond well to stimulant medication." Another problem often encountered in these situations is that many physicians are not skilled in determining appropriate dosage levels, given the age and size of a child. These physicians may also be less comfortable trying different dosages or even alternate stimulants if the initial dosage and choice does not work effectively.

This advocacy and consulting process can become even more difficult when it involves referring an ADHD adult for medication. Many physicians, as well as some psychiatrists, are simply not willing to prescribe stimulant medication for adult ADHD patients. In these cases, having a psychiatrist in a referral network is invaluable. For managed care patients whose coverage may not include the psychiatrists with whom you typically work, the psychiatrist can provide the initial medical evaluation and prescription and follow the patient medically for the first month; then your psychiatrist can make a written referral explaining the diagnosis and medication to the patient's primary care physician and pass the patient on to her or him. In most cases the primary care physician is comfortable following the psychiatrist's recommendations.

Many ADHD children and adolescents, whether or not they have been diagnosed, are in therapy with clinicians for other symptomatic problems—often conduct disorders and occasionally depression. In such cases the therapist making the ADHD diagnosis will need to consult with, and at times educate, the therapist treating the child or adolescent for behavioral manifestations of the ADHD disorder. Not all therapists are open to another professional offering a "new" diagnosis for their patients. Naturally, it is important to support an individual's ongoing therapy. Some of these therapists, when they learn of the ADHD diagnosis, will acknowledge their lack of expertise in this area and refer the case to us to work with for a period of time. In most of these situations we will gladly work with the referring therapist in a collaborative or consulting relationship, unless he or she prefers to exit from the treatment process. Sometimes we will provide family therapy for the parents and the ADHD child, while the referring therapist continues to provide individual therapy for the child. In other cases we may provide marital therapy for the ADHD adult and spouse, while one or both remain in individual therapy with other clinicians. Many ADHD adults may already be in individual therapy for comorbid conditions. They or their spouse may be working with a psychiatrist for depression or receiving antidepressant medications from a primary care physician. Here again, the diagnosing therapist can become both a coordinator and an advocate to make sure that the ADHD patient receives the most effective treatment from the professionals involved.

Advocacy in Legal Matters

We have become involved with this more specialized adjunctive role as a result of years of experience doing custodial evaluations in court settings. We do not recommend this role for therapists unless they have prior experience working with legal matters and testifying in court. That said, it can be a highly effective advocacy role.

Most of the legal cases in which we have participated have involved ADHD adolescents whose conduct has propelled them into delinquent activities based occasionally on destructive and reactive behaviors, but more often on impulsivity. Examples of these impulsive behaviors include spray painting graffiti on a neighbor's wall, setting fire to a box in a vacant field near a school, showing a pocket knife to a friend in class, or taking the parents' car at 2 A.M. for a drive around the neighborhood with a friend. One 12-year-old boy was banned from Boy Scouts because during a meeting he inhaled propane gas, blew it out of his mouth, and lit it with matches, proudly displaying his ability as a human flamethrower. Many ADHD children and adolescents, particularly the hyperactive–impulsive type, have experienced a broad range of problematic behaviors that carry more serious consequences as they get older. The "innocent" pranks from their childhood now yield sobering legal consequences for them as adolescents and young adults.

In this context we often talk with, and try to educate, juvenile probation officers about the role ADHD can play in an adolescent's problematic behaviors. The issue here is not to use the ADHD diagnosis as an excuse for the child's behaviors but to help the probation officers, the courts, and often the parents "fit the punishment to the crime."

One of the authors (CAE) recently received a call from the father of an ADHD child, whom he had worked with as a fifth-grader. The child was now in the ninth grade and had been arrested for displaying a knife in school. He was not arrested until after the police interviewed his older sister at their home. The father was not present and the sister dramatized the situation by telling the officers that her brother was often intimidating and violent toward her.

It turned out that the adolescent had taken a pocket knife to school to show off to his friends, despite having been told not to do so by his father and the school counselor. In his evaluation the probation officer indicated that he believed that the student was a potential gang member and a danger to his family. When the therapist met with the student and his parents, it was apparent that the boy was still quite immature and feeling somewhat overwhelmed by his entrance into high school. It was also apparent that he still displayed considerable hyperactive and impulsive symptoms. The parents acknowledged that he had not been taking Ritalin for several years. The student was referred back to his physician, and the prescription for Ritalin was continued. His impulsive behaviors and conflicts with his sister settled down within the week. The therapist assured the probation officer that, with the medication, the youngster's impulsive behaviors should improve and that he was not a threat to his family or the community. The parents also explained to the probation officer that the sister's prior report was exaggerated and that she was now sorry for getting her brother into further trouble. The probation officer required that the student attend five therapy sessions over the next 2 months, "just to make sure everything will be all right."

A more dramatic advocacy case involved the issue of "corporal punishment" by a foster parent toward an 8-year-old ADHD child. One of the authors (CAE) became involved in this case as a favor to an attorney.

The foster parent had been charged with child abuse. She was a 45-year-old woman who had cared for hundreds of foster children on both a long-term and an acute basis. She had recently adopted a 3-year-old girl who had previously been placed with her as a foster child. She had no history of punitive or physically harmful behaviors toward any of the prior foster placements. The 8-year-old had been with her for about 2 months. There was a suspicion that he had been sexually abused by a parent or prior childcare worker. He had been seen by a child psychiatrist on two occasions because of his use of sexual language with another foster child and a student at his school. The psychiatrist had diagnosed the child as "possible ADHD" but had not followed up by medicating the child. The teacher and foster mother described the child as often uncooperative, unruly, restless, impulsive, and confrontational with other students.

One afternoon the foster mother was called to the school by the principal to remove the child because he had started a fight with another student and refused to stay in the principal's office. The foster mother picked up the child, who was reluctant to leave the school building with her, took him by his arm, and left the school. On the way down the steps of the school the child tried to pull away from the foster mother and, at the same time, knocked her purse to the ground. The foster mother "swatted" the child with her open hand on his behind. The principal was watching them out of her window and reported the incident to the state's child protective program. The mother was charged with "abuse," but the charges were later dropped. However, the state was now attempting to remove her foster care license and to remove her recently adopted 3-year-old daughter. CAE testified as an expert on ADHD and on behalf of the foster mother, reviewing the child's symptomatic behaviors as reported by both the foster mother and the school, explaining the preliminary diagnosis of ADHD by the psychiatrist, and supporting the fact that without medication this would have been a difficult child to manage and that the mild physical punishment issued by the mother was not excessive.

In court we debated the "fine line" between supporting physical punishment of ADHD children, which we do not, and recognizing a foster mother's frustration in managing an unmedicated ADHD child. Unfortunately, because of the state's rules regarding "no hitting," the foster mother lost the case. The court ruled that her physical response to the child was based on "anger and frustration" and was not a clear incident of punishment. The state revoked her license and took away her young adopted child.

THE PSYCHOEDUCATIONAL ROLE

The efficacy of psychoeducational approaches as sole interventions for a variety of clinical disorders is a current topic of debate in the mental health field. There are a number of groups, for example, who believe that marital education can be more effective for conflicted couples than traditional couples therapy. In truth, most therapists provide some degree of educational material in their ongoing therapeutic activities. This may take the form of information about diagnoses, medication, developmental stages, career issues, or even financial management. In our practices working with family, marital, and child cases, we often find that psychoeducational approaches helpful in our therapeutic roles. Most often, we impart information about parenting and child management, mate selection, marital roles and communication, family hierarchies, intergenerational dynamics and boundaries, and balancing parental and spousal roles.

The therapist working with ADHD families has a necessary psychoeducational role. Due to the neurobiological nature of the disorder and its chronicity throughout an individual's life experiences, family members need to learn about its etiology, the extent of symptomatology, and the nature of its effects, just as they would if their child had diabetes or a congenital heart defect. ADHD symptoms can be so intrusive and compelling that they evoke more dramatic and destructive responses than might be seen in a family with a physically disabled child. Thus education regarding the disorder becomes a crucial ingredient in successful therapeutic interventions. In families where the ADHD child has not been diagnosed, there is considerably more destructive scapegoating of the child, as well as more severe interactional dysfunctions throughout the entire family system.

We believe that this psychoeducational role needs to become a clearly defined aspect of the clinician's work with ADHD families. It should be defined in the early stages of the evaluation and treatment, and it should be available to all members of both the nuclear and extended families as needed. In the following chapters we will discuss how we implement this psychoeducational role in the context of family therapy. It involves much more than simply handing the family a pamphlet to read, as one might do for patients with depression or anxiety disorders. Some of the ingredients of this psychoeducational role that we utilize therapeutically are listed in Table 3.1.

The therapist's role as educator and expert on ADHD as a disorder must be clear and direct. It often involves explaining to family members such issues as the following:

1. The nature and range of the symptomatology.
2. The practical effects of the symptoms on everyday life.
3. The ingredients of an evaluation.
4. The role of potential testing.
5. The disorder's etiology and potential for intergenerational transmission.
6. The treatment plan.
7. The need for interprofessional collaboration.
8. The potential effectiveness of medication.
9. The types and chemical effects of medication.
10. The media's attack on stimulant medications and how that might affect their attitudes regarding the use of medication.
11. The potential advocacy roles in school or work settings.
12. The focus of the individual and family therapy sessions.

The therapist working with ADHD patients will need to continue to be up to date on the latest research regarding new medications and treatment approaches. But in addition to this, the therapist will need to learn to function in this educational role at many differing levels. For example:

TABLE 3.1. Psychoeducational Information Provided for the ADHD Family

ADHD: Facts and ramifications
  Summary and interpretation of recent theories and research on the origins of ADHD
  Discussion of the bioneurological effects
  Discussion of the potential for intergenerational transmission
  Identification of possible comorbid disorders
  Exploration of the psychological components of ADHD in terms of self-esteem and self-confidence
  Identification of the effects of ADHD at differing stages of the life cycle, including adulthood

The diagnostic process
  Discussion of the diagnostic process
  Differentiation of ADHD from other disorders
  Identification of the cluster of cognitive and behavioral symptoms
  Differentiation of the three diagnostic categories: hyperactivity–impulsivity, inattentive, and combined
  Discussion of the role of testing

The treatment process
  Exploration of the role of other professionals and the use of consultants
  Exploration of the possible role and expectations of medication

Advocacy issues
  Discussion of advocacy role in the schools
  If needed, discussion of legal issues and possible courses of action

The therapist may need to sit on the floor of a playroom and explain what ADHD is and might mean to a 9-year-old girl.

The therapist may need to find a way to convince a resistant and reactive adolescent not only that he has ADHD but that medication and educational accommodations can really help him become more successful in school.

The therapist may need to explain the ADHD disorder carefully and answer pointed questions from skeptical or disbelieving parents or grandparents.

The therapist may need to assemble an entire family of grandparents, parents, adolescents, and young children in order to make sure that all the members of the system have the same, accurate information about the ADHD adolescent's disorder.

Parents, siblings, and involved grandparents all deserve to be educated about their family member's disorder. The therapeutic issue here is that by making available this information to the entire family, each member can begin to view the ADHD individual's symptoms and behaviors with greater understanding and objectivity.

We have found that for older grade school children, adolescents, and adults with ADHD, this educational information—which explains and even labels their struggles as a known and treatable disorder—is often experienced as a *relief* and provides them with *a sense of hope.*

In a family meeting that included an 11-year-old ADHD brother, his 13- and 15-year-old sisters, both parents, and a grandmother, the therapist (SVE) carefully explained the meaning of ADHD and gave examples of how the disorder affects an entire family. Before he was halfway through his discussion the 15-year-old sister began to cry uncontrollable. The therapist glanced over and noticed that the mother and grandmother were also beginning to cry. The sister finally said that she was "so sorry" for the way she had talked about and treated her brother all of these years. She said, "I always thought he was just a brat who hated me and the family." The grandmother, a retired elementary school teacher, said, "If we had only known, we would have never been so angry and punitive." The mother needed 10 minutes before she could compose herself and "apologize" to her son. The father, who was later found to have ADHD himself, expressed his sense of guilt and admitted "how much of myself" he had always seen in his son. This family feedback meeting took place about 4 weeks into the therapeutic process, just after the son's test results were received. This meeting, which addressed only informational issues about ADHD and never even touched upon the broader family dynamics, became dramatically healing for everyone.

The other area of psychoeducational work with ADHD families is that of parent education, which we will discuss in more detail in Chapter 6. Parent education involves the direct instruction of parents on specific child management strategies and skills as related to age-appropriate expectations of their ADHD child or adolescent. It may involve recommendations of supplemental reading or homework assignments to provide basic and practical tools for the parents. We have found that it is most effective in helping parents (1) learn how to provide more structure and consistency in behavioral expectations (which is central to working with an ADHD child); (2) learn appropriate types and levels of consequences based on the nature of the behavioral problems and the age of their child; and (3) gain a better sense of control and empowerment as parents, particularly if they have been struggling for years with disruptive ADHD behaviors. One study suggested that parent education should focus on training parents to be "case managers" and organizers of their ADHD child's social environment and competencies (Cousins & Weiss, 1993). Parent education can become a critically important resource for all parents of ADHD children or adolescents; however, there are limitations to its effectiveness. We have observed, as have others (Estrada & Pinsof, 1995; Pisterman et al., 1989, 1992), that parent education cannot effectively change the basic symptoms of hyperactivity and inattention in an ADHD child or adolescent. Of course, the results of outcome studies involving parent education improve considerably when the ADHD children have been stabilized on stimulant medications (Henry, 1987). Studies also report that, while parent education can reduce the severity of the ADHD child's disruptive behaviors, the primary benefit for the parents appears to be in decreased stress and improved confidence and self-esteem regarding their parenting (Anastopoulos et al., 1993; Erhardt & Baker, 1990).

In the next chapter, on further clinical assessment and interventions, we will discuss more specifically how these various roles evolve for the therapist.

APPENDIX 3.1. SAMPLE LETTER TO A SCHOOL
ON BEHALF OF A FAMILY

Ms. Joan Smith
Principal, River Bend Elementary School

Dear Ms. Smith:

One of your students, Elizabeth Johnson (6th grade, Ms. Williams's class), has been referred to me recently regarding her disruptive behaviors at home and at school. After talking briefly with her teacher and compiling a history with her parents, I believe that there is a possibility that she may have ADHD and/or underlying cognitive processing difficulties. In addition to her difficulties of disrupting her class and her inattentiveness, she also reports problems in the areas of completing tests in the allotted time, expressing her thoughts in written reports, and understanding and recalling verbal requests and assignments.

I would like to request your assistance in testing Elizabeth to help rule out underlying processing deficits or other underlying learning disabilities, and/or ADHD, and her potential need for special education services. I would recommend that she be administered the WISC-III and both parts of the WJ-R. Please feel free to call me if I can provide you with additional information.

Sincerely,

Sandra Volgy Everett, PHD

APPENDIX 3.2. POTENTIAL ACCOMMODATIONS PREPARED FOR A HIGH SCHOOL 504 MEETING

Proposed Accommodations for Joseph Hill, 9th grade

Diagnosis: ADHD

Algebra: Primary difficulties in areas of differentiating details such as numbers and signs, committing more errors when rushed, lowest scores on WISC were in Coding and Digit Span.

1. Provide additional time on tests and examinations, and/or
2. Develop alternative testing formats

English: Joseph enjoys reading but has problems with grammar, punctuation, sentence and paragraph structure, spelling, and proofreading.

3. Written assignments to be graded for content rather than grammar
4. Provide alternative formats for testing—multiple choice is more realistic than essays
5. Provide alternatives in vocabulary tests—use shorter lists for memorization and possibly matching rather than filling in the blanks for sentence completion

6. Develop alternative assignments and testing for grammar (Joseph says "I can see that something is wrong but I can't fix it.")
7. Allow additional time for assignments and tests that require reading lengthy passages

General Issues for Other Classes:

8. Whenever possible, replace written reports and essays with alternative assignments or tests
9. Grade all written reports and essays for content and not grammar
10. Assist his organizational needs with written outlines and assignments whenever possible
11. Recognize that Joseph's cursive writing is difficult for him and hard to read—accept printing with extra time allowed in class assignments and tests
12. Develop creative formats to review Joseph's true knowledge on a subject, avoid requesting him to integrate multiple concepts—particularly in a time-limited format
13. Anticipate preparing Joseph's application in advance for approval to take the SAT next semester in an alternate setting

APPENDIX 3.3. POTENTIAL ACCOMMODATIONS PREPARED FOR A GRADE SCHOOL 504 MEETING

Proposed Accommodations for Mary Hill, 4th grade

Diagnosis: ADHD with associated depressive symptoms

Specific Cognitive Deficits (based on history and testing):

1. Visual processing
2. Auditory processing
3. Short-term memory
4. Written language

General Symptoms:

1. Difficulty retaining auditory instructions
2. Difficulty processing and recording instructions and information written on the board
3. Difficulty organizing cognitive information and expressing it in writing

4. Difficulty retaining general information and assignments from morning to afternoon, or from day-to-day

Language Arts:

- Provide handouts and written instruction for classroom activities and homework assignments
- Potential need for remedial work in the mechanics of written language
- Develop alternative methods to test for spelling skills, such as verbal, recognition, and comparative methods
- Provide additional assistance in study skills to enhance memorization

Physical Education:

- Student and parents need to make sure appropriate clothing is always available at school

Social Studies:

- Provide outlines and/or notes on lectures
- Identify a student from whom she can compare notes from class
- Provide homework assignments in writing

Science:

- Provide alternatives to written reports, such as verbal presentations, outlines, etc.
- Provide additional time for essay tests
- Provide alternative test formats to essays whenever possible

Math:

- Consider seating location to minimize distractions
- Provide handouts of classroom activities rather than relying on problems written on the board
- Provide additional time for testing

Teachers need to assist Mary in developing a specific checklist for each class to help her organize and remember to complete and turn in assignments.

4

Assessing ADHD in the Intergenerational Family System

As marital and family therapy educators, we have observed that the greatest leap clinicians must make to be effective in working with family problems is to learn to look at the *bigger picture* and the overall life of a family system rather than just the symptoms presented by individuals. Once the therapist learns to look for patterns and solutions in the larger intergenerational system, the questions that he or she asks clinically become very different than those utilized in treating individuals in isolation from their families. We believe strongly that the most effective way to understand and treat ADHD is within the context of the ADHD member's family system.

The research and literature on ADHD focuses primarily on the symptoms and behaviors of the identified ADHD child or adult. Secondary sources focus on behavioral and educational management issues for parents and teachers. While most experts in this field acknowledge that the ADHD child's family environment has an impact on behavior and psychological adjustment, few resources are available, either theoretically or clinically, to help the therapist identify and track the impact of ADHD on a family system's members and life cycle.

Moreover, the family's reciprocal attitudes and responses toward the ADHD member influence both the ADHD individual's level of symptomatic behaviors and the severity of potential comorbid disorders. For example, an ADHD adolescent's educational and behavioral struggles may cause reciprocal responses of frustration, anger, and embarrassment by the parents and siblings. These reactions may well intensify the adolescent's frustrations, impulsivity, and reactivity, and produce additional symptoms of anxiety, depression, or a conduct disorder, which in turn impact the whole family, and so on.

The family system also provides a wealth of resources that can be used—often with dramatic results—in the treatment process. For example, a sibling's relationship with an ADHD sister or brother can be developed around activities such as computer games or sports in such a way as to enhance support and repair self-esteem problems. A grandparent's role can be developed to provide additional attention for an ADHD child through activities such as reading to the child or providing help with his or her homework to restore self-confidence. Utilizing the interactive resources of a family can create more lasting changes than simply sending the hyperactive child off to play soccer so that her or his energy level can be dissipated (the latter, of course, may help too).

We are frequently asked, by both colleagues and parents, to run groups for ADHD children and adolescents. While we find that certain support groups for ADHD children can be helpful, we believe that we can be more helpful and can promote more constructive changes by working with the child in the context of her or his family dynamics. Similarly, with ADHD adults, we believe that the treatment of choice is a combination of individual, marital, and family therapy.

To enhance effective assessment and treatment, the therapist needs to recognize the reciprocal interaction between the family dynamics and the ADHD in one or multiple family members, *and* the variability of these patterns through each life-cycle stage. In this chapter we will discuss the family dynamics within the nuclear family and across intergenerational family systems. In the next chapter we will discuss tracking these interactive patterns through the life cycle.

In this chapter we will:

1. Identify family systems concepts that help explain the influence of ADHD.
2. Discuss the use of family genograms.
3. Track the influence of ADHD across three family generations.
4. Define seven systemic dynamics of ADHD families.
5. Identify 11 factors in the intergenerational transmission of ADHD.

A FAMILY SYSTEMS PERSPECTIVE ON ADHD

The family system is a unique and complex "organism" with remarkable resources for accommodation and survival. Despite alarm raised

in the United States about the 50% divorce rate and pessimistic fore-
casts regarding the future of the family, family life continues to be central to most individuals' daily experiences. Despite high levels of
acrimony during the divorce process, postdivorce and binuclear family systems develop stable patterns of interaction to provide their children with safe and nurturing environments. Other family systems that
struggle with a member's chronic disability or a diagnosis of terminal
cancer also find resources to rebalance themselves, provide support,
and survive. Often the support for families in crisis, both emotional
and financial, is provided by intergenerational resources such as parents, grandparents, or adult siblings. While this interactional network,
which might span several generations, can provide support and assistance, it can also become part of dysfunctional patterns and behaviors
that are experienced throughout the family system.

For example, a family system with an acutely depressed parent
must find a way to remain in balance to continue to function on a daily
basis. The family system, as a living organism, is motion, and the directions and patterns of the movements are made in response to changes,
both internally or externally, that may create an imbalance. The presence
of a depressed parent does not always elicit a kind and understanding
response from other family members. Some family systems may push
the depressed parent aside, trying to continue everyday activities by
denying or avoiding this individual's pain. Other family systems may
engage in an ongoing power struggle with the depressed parent, hoping
to "argue" the member out of his or her depression. In some family systems the nonsymptomatic parent may internalize the partner's symptoms and display depression herself or himself. This depressed
member's role in the hierarchy of the system also defines the system's
response. When the primary caretaker becomes depressed, the system
experiences more chaos until another member can assume the leadership role. These rebalancings may be provided by a parent, a "parentified" child, or an extended family member.

When an ADHD child is present in a family, the parents must
struggle, similarly, to create a stable balance for the family and accommodate to the intrusive and maddening symptoms of their child's disorder. This balancing act, which we often describe as such to families,
is called "homeostasis" and is present in all family systems. *Homeostasis* is the ongoing process by which a family struggles to remain in a
working balance despite disruptive or dysfunctional influences. Just as
a thermostat functions to keep a room's temperature hovering around
72 degrees, homeostasis functions in the ADHD family's activities and
behaviors to maintain them within a stable range. For example, an
ADHD child's impulsive and intrusive behaviors do not occur in a

vacuum: they elicit reciprocal responses from all members. These behaviors may push the family into chaos, evidenced by yelling parents and fighting siblings. Some members may react to the disruption with anger and resentment and others with control or withdrawal. While all members will react, their responses may push the system into further imbalance (and loss of homeostasis). Some families have the resources of a parent or a hierarchical structure to restore the balance, but other families enter therapy in a state of chaos that may have been present for several years.

These examples illustrate the concepts of *circularity* and the *reciprocity* within a family system. All events, actions, and behaviors experienced by one member will also be experienced throughout the family system. The more serious or dramatic the event, the more widespread the effect throughout the system. Like the circular ripples made by a single pebble dropped into a still pond, the family event "ripples" create splashes "when they reach the rocks" (individual family members) on the shore. The ADHD child's disruptive behaviors, experienced in differing ways by all the family members, elicit reactions by these members as well as from their intergenerational and social networks. The clinician needs to recognize and understand how these circular and reciprocal responses are influenced by the presence of an ADHD member. A potential scenario may appear as the following:

An inattentive ADHD child chronically forgets his mother's instructions to take his books to his room after school, which provokes her frustrated attempts to organize or control his behaviors. The frustrated mother becomes impatient and snaps at the other children. The husband arrives home from work to find that he has become the target of his wife's frustrations during the day, and even of her life in general. The grandparents, who had been saving money to send their inattentive grandchild to college, become angry at their son and daughter-in-law for poor parenting and cannot understand how the parents can allow the child to forget to turn in assignments and to be on the verge of failing. The teacher tells the frustrated parents that she just cannot get their son's attention and he is falling behind in reading and math. The school principal tells the parents and the frustrated teacher that the child may be required to repeat the school year because he is immature and lazy.

For the reader less familiar with family systems theory, it is helpful to visualize the larger intergenerational system as a series of *subsystems* that define both the *hierarchy* and the *membership* of each group (see Figure 4.1). Visualizing this structure will make it easier for the therapist to recognize and isolate both the source of certain symptoms and the manner in which they have spread through the system.

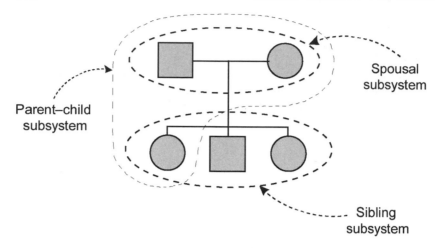

FIGURE 4.1. Family subsystems.

Since the ADHD family member is most often a child or adolescent, the behavioral symptoms will originate in the *sibling subsystem*. The hierarchy expected in a family system suggests that the decision-making power occurs within the *spousal subsystem* since the adult roles are defined here. The *parent–child subsystem* defines the interactional roles, and to some extent, the authority between the adults and the children. The *intergenerational system* identifies other important "players" in the family system, such as grandparents, aunts, and uncles, who may provide support or intrusive disruptions to the family.

These subsystems provide the clinician with an important range of data for both assessment and treatment. For example, it is important to understand how the ADHD child's symptoms are both experienced by and responded to reciprocally by each sibling. There may be an older brother who distances or isolates himself from his younger ADHD brother because he is frustrated or embarrassed by this brother's disruptions and impulsivity. An older sister in the family may be more sympathetic and willing to try to be friends with her ADHD brother. But a younger brother may excel at provoking and overstimulating the ADHD brother, often leading to physical confrontations. The younger non-ADHD brother may gain recognition from his parents as a victim or may simply feel that negative attention is better than no attention at all. If the clinician is not aware of these dynamics within the sibling subsystem, her or his clinical interventions toward restructuring parental roles or enhancing positive interaction among the siblings may fail.

The hierarchy in many ADHD families may not be clearly defined. The power within a family may actually be usurped by the disruptive behaviors of the ADHD child. Many parents report "feeling powerless" or "lacking control." Siblings report being angry or jealous about the attention (although primarily negative) that their ADHD sibling receives. If the therapist focuses solely on instructing the parents in better management skills and fails to recognize that the ADHD child has more power than the parents, interventions will fail.

In contrast to working with children, which involves parent–child interactions, the therapist working with ADHD adults must address both their *spousal* and their *parent–child subsystems.* Their symptoms of impulsivity, reactivity, and forgetfulness will elicit reciprocal responses from their spouses that range from perplexity to rage. Of course, these symptoms also effect the adult's parenting role as well as the children's responses, which may range from confusion to anger.

For example, the spouse of an inattentive ADHD adult often reports feeling exasperated by their partner's inability to remember instructions or even conversations that occurred the same day. The spouse eventually interprets her or his ADHD partner's inattention as "disinterest" or "rejection." When the ADHD parent forgets remarks or requests, the children feel confused and frustrated, and, seeing their parent as unreliable, their hurt feelings may escalate into anger and disrespect. Since the parent's inattention can vary according to time and subjects, children and spouses may conclude that it is intentional and willful. These circular and reciprocal experiences clearly create conflict, misunderstanding, and often chaos throughout the family's experiences.

It is also important for the clinician to be able to recognize (and visualize) a family system's *boundaries,* the imaginary lines that define who is within the system and who is outside of the system (see Figure 4.2). Boundaries circumscribe the nuclear family system as well as each of the subsystems that we have identified. These boundaries are like territorial markers because they serve to define and protect the system. They differ in shapes and degrees, and are characterized as *rigid, flexible, diffuse, open,* or *closed.*

Diffuse boundaries offer families little protection from external intrusions and input, as well as offering limited definitions for its members (Nichols & Everett, 1987). These systems may be marked by internal confusion or chaos due to unwanted intrusions by grandparents or community sources. In contrast, *closed boundaries* circumscribe the family tightly, resulting in social and family-of-origin isolation and the restriction of external feedback. It is difficult for members to successfully separate and leave families with closed boundaries. The ideal

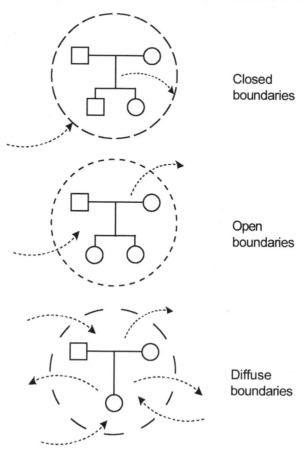

Closed
boundaries

Open
boundaries

Diffuse
boundaries

FIGURE 4.2. Family systems boundaries.

is *open boundaries,* which allow a greater exchange of feedback between the family and its environment but also offer enough definition to protect the family without isolating its members. It is helpful to think of these boundaries as existing on a continuum: the open boundaries would appear toward the middle, the diffuse and closed boundaries would exist toward either end. The healthier functioning families tend to have boundaries closer to the center of the continuum.

Boundaries also have the properties of being rigid or flexible. *Rigid boundaries* do not adjust readily to changes in the environment or to new events. *Flexible boundaries* can open and close according to the needs of the family and relative changes that occur in the environment.

In general, healthy families display more flexible boundaries, but all family systems benefit from continual adjustment of their boundaries. For example, a young adult couple, recently married, may need to "close" and tighten their system's boundaries temporarily so that they can protect their new relationship, provide privacy for their relationship from external intrusions, and allow time for bonding. However, this couple may not want to keep these boundaries rigidly closed unless they are protecting themselves from highly intrusive parents. When their first child in born, the couple will want to open and relax their boundaries more to allow the grandparents to support their parenting and interact with their grandchild. But if the grandparents become too intrusive, the couple will need to exercise the flexibility of their boundaries to close them temporarily to protect the privacy of their family life. These concepts of subsystems and boundaries are important to assessing family dynamics and developing clinical strategies.

Stressors and environmental changes are experienced and shared by all members of the family system. These stressors spread quickly throughout several generations of a family such that the original stress experienced by one member is experienced soon by other members across several generations. Often the stress becomes identified with one member who assumes a certain stereotyped role within the family referred to as a *family scapegoat.*

In the family system the scapegoat, identified in early family systems theory literature (Ackerman, 1958; Bell & Vogel, 1961), receives and carries (and often acts out) the stress, anger, and unhappiness that is experienced within the family. In many clinical situations the scapegoated child carries the unhappiness of the marital partners. When the spouses designate a child as the source of all their discord, the marital relationship may return, temporarily, to a level of stability, with the spouses' conflict and anger somewhat diffused. But, if the scapegoated child's behaviors improve, such that he or she can no longer be blamed for causing trouble, or if the child is removed from the household, the marriage immediately begins to display stress again—until another child is scapegoated.

The scapegoat may be labeled as such (by projection) for a variety of reasons—for example, she or he looks different physically, may be the eldest or youngest member, or displays a more emotionally reactive temperament than other members of the family. In families where one member, particularly a child, is a chronic source of stress and disruption, that child typically is targeted as the scapegoat. As a result of this identification, the scapegoat, through the reciprocal interactions of the family, assumes this role and develops an internal identity that is consistent with the family image. This role is often enacted not only within the family but also at school and in the wide community, and may follow the child into her or his young adult life.

Many ADHD children experience this role of scapegoat in their families. (Many undiagnosed ADHD adults will also have played this role in their families of origin.) The child's disruptive behavior demands time, energy, and resources from parents as well as siblings, grandparents, and teachers. The family's continual response to these behaviors provokes frustration and eventually anger from the caregivers. Soon the ADHD child is labeled, either literally or in the caregivers' minds, as a "problem child," a "screwup," "lazy," or "retarded." Comparative studies of parents with and without ADHD children consistently confirm that the parents of ADHD children display lower self-esteem, greater negativity about their child's behaviors, higher personal and parenting stress, and a sense that their child's behavior negatively affected other areas of their lives (Anastopoulous et al., 1992; Baker & McCall, 1995; Baldwin et al., 1995; Culbertson & Silovsky, 1996; Johnson, 1996; Johnson & Behrenz, 1993).

The assigned role and identity of an ADHD child in a family, whether or not the child has been diagnosed, spreads quickly among all family members, as well as the network of teachers and caregivers. The parents' own view of themselves shifts to that of "parents with a problem child or an ADHD child"; the identity of the siblings now becomes that of "having a disruptive or an ADHD brother or sister," the identity of the teacher becomes that of "having a problem child or ADHD student in the classroom." These dynamics, focused on a scapegoated ADHD child, can be detrimental to the parents' marriage, the siblings' interaction and bonding, and the entire family's quality of life.

Justin, a 10-year-old fifth-grade student, was referred to one of the authors (SVE) due to continual fighting with his siblings and increasing failures in school. The therapist could sense from the initial meeting with his parents that he had been intensely scapegoated. They expressed anger at him, disgust at his behaviors, and spoke in demeaning tones. After an initial individual meeting with Justin, it was decided to see him with his siblings rather than with his parents. It was felt that the parents would continue to scapegoat him in a parent–child meeting and the therapist wished to block (avoid) that dynamic at the beginning of therapy. Seeing the child with siblings often diffuses the parents' anger and blaming and helps us experience a broader sense of the child's role by viewing the sibling subsystem. Justin was seen with his two siblings: a 14-year-old sister, Joan, and a 7-year-old brother, Billy.

At the beginning of the session Billy spoke first and for the entire family.

He chastised Justin for a long list of disruptive behaviors: "embarrassing the family at school by fighting," "going into my room and taking my things," "picking on our sister," "pushing me into a wall last summer," and "making Mommy and Daddy fight all the time." As the therapist tried to interrupt Billy's attack, Justin was withdrawing and had pushed his chair back from the circle of chairs in the office. He was looking down at the floor. Joan was quiet at first but soon picked up the attack on Justin by saying that she wished that he was not even her brother. When the therapist was able to divert the attention away from Justin's behaviors, it was clear that any closeness or respect for Justin as a brother had been damaged seriously many years earlier by the family's failure to recognize and better manage Justin's disruptive behaviors. Justin was later diagnosed as ADHD. It was clear that these symptomatic behaviors had targeted him as the family's scapegoat.

THE INTRUSION OF ADHD ACROSS THREE FAMILY GENERATIONS

Because of the complexity of ADHD as a bioneurological and psychiatric disorder, clinicians, as well as school counselors who may only see the child (not the whole family), need to recognize the influence of the disorder throughout the "bigger picture" of the intergenerational family system. This means that the therapist must always be on the lookout for *other family members who display ADHD symptoms but who have not been diagnosed.* These may include parents, siblings, aunts and uncles, or grandparents.

Geneticists and anthropologists, who study and track biological or behavioral phenomena across generations, have technical procedures for "mapping" the locations of the participants and significant patterns across time. They create diagrams called *genograms.* Family therapists value the use of genograms because they provide a visual picture of the family's structure and organization, hierarchy and patterns of interaction, and the location of certain themes or stressors. As we will illustrate with ADHD families, these patterns can span many generations (see Figure 4.3).

The therapist needs to be able to recognize and track both subtle and dramatic intergenerational patterns and themes. For example, a marital case (non-ADHD) displayed four generations of females who exhibited primary decision-making power and control within their respective nuclear families. These females devalued, fairly blatantly, male roles. By using a genogram in our assessment, we were able to ask broader questions about the history of gender perceptions and roles. The wife reported that her maternal grandfather "slept in a shed

Generations

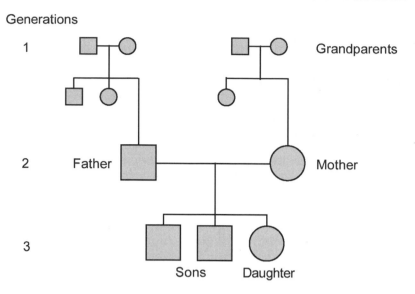

FIGURE 4.3. A three-generational genogram.

behind the house" and that her own father had "slept on the back porch" for most of her youth. She indicated that she had slept in her mother's bed until she was 13 years old, and that since her marriage she had often asked her husband to "sleep on the couch." The drama of this intergenerational pattern continued in that her 8-year-old daughter was allowed to sleep with her (this was one of the reasons the father was asked to leave the bedroom). However, the 5-year-old son was never allowed into the mother's bed. This marriage displayed poor communication, conflicted parenting, depression in the wife, and anger display by the husband. The genogram aided us in mapping the broadly transmitted intergenerational dynamics and helped us recognize and make plans to interrupt historical attitudes and patterns. When we showed the wife our genogram, which clearly illustrated the strikingly similar patterns of her own family with those of her parents and grandparents, she became tearful and acknowledged that she had always felt that "something was not right" but could never "see the whole picture." She and her husband made immediate changes to correct the problems and eventually relocated several hundred miles from the powerful negative influences of her family.

Bioneurological research (reviewed in Chapter 1) tends to support the intergenerational transmission of ADHD. We have noted that other studies and clinical observations have not effectively addressed the notion that parallel emotional and interactional patterns are also transmitted intergenerationally through the ADHD family system. We encourage clinicians, in order to learn to think in terms of the "bigger picture," to learn to create and use genograms in their work with ADHD. One may start by drawing a diagram of her or his own family of origin using the symbols in Figure 4.3. This is how we teach our clinical students to become acquainted with thinking in terms of family systems and translating systemic patterns into a visual picture. Move from the drawing of a genogram of your own family to that of a marital case with which you are working.

In drawing the genogram, try to fit the knowledge you possess into a visual scheme. Draw the families of origin of each spouse. Do you know the ordinal position of each member and where they fit into their sibling subsystems? Do you know which of their parents are living or deceased? Write on your diagram the causes of death of other family members. Can you identify those who may have been treated for depression or alcoholism? Did any of the siblings drop out of high school? How many completed college? How many divorces have occurred?

It will become apparent through this exercise that *to draw a thorough family genogram the therapist must ask broader systemic questions and recognize larger interactional patterns.* The therapist needs to learn to look beyond the individual symptoms of a disruptive or ADHD child. This is the "leap" that we mentioned earlier: *to reconceptualize symptoms from a systems perspective by thinking in terms of broad patterns of interaction that may occur within and across nuclear and intergenerational subsystems.*

We have created a sample genogram (Figure 4.4) to illustrate a pattern of transmission of ADHD across five generations. The ADHD son, labeled # 4 for his generation, is the presenting patient. We have designed this genogram, for illustration purposes, to reflect the transmission of ADHD through the *males* in the family. The ADHD is transmitted from the father (3), to the child (4). The father's ADHD is present symptomatically in the parenting to his two children (4 and 4a) and in his marital relationship (3c). The genogram also illustrates that the father's own ADHD symptoms were present, probably in a disruptive manner, during his childhood and with his two sisters (3a and 3b).

Looking at the intergenerational picture, this father, may have inherited the ADHD from his father (2), the paternal grandfather of the identified child (4). This father's traits would have also been present in his parenting of his children, numbers 3, 3a, and 3b; in his marriage (2c), and historical in his role with his brothers (2a and 2b). Clinical data beyond this generation is much harder to confirm with most fami-

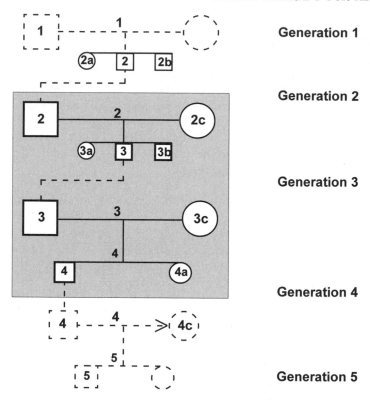

FIGURE 4.4. The transmission of ADHD across five generations.

lies. Hypothetically (see the dotted arrow from 1), we can suggest that the ADHD came from the great-grandfather (1). (For readers who wish to speculate beyond this first generation, we refer them to Hartmann, 1993, who suggested that ADHD behaviors may have been useful survival traits for the early hunter in primitive cultures, less useful in terms of survival to the agriculturalist, and not useful at all in modern urban cultures.)

Looking ahead, the ADHD child's (4) symptoms will likely occur throughout his life experiences: in his role as a son, in his relationship with his siblings, in his future mate selection (4c) and subsequent marital dynamics, and in his future parenting. The ADHD may also be transmitted to his son (5). We have oversimplified this model for illustration purposes, but the potential patterns are realistic. If males 2, 3, and 4 were diagnosed with ADHD, predominantly hyperactive–impulsive type, it would not be unusual to find ADHD, predominantly inattentive type, in sisters 3b and 4a. The clinical evidence and influence of other ADHD family members becomes clear through the development of a genogram.

If we expand this genogram by adding emotional and behavioral traits, in addition to the ADHD component, the clinical problems become more complex (see Figure 4.5). In the nuclear system of husband (3), wife (3c), and children (4 and 4a), there is an overlay of circular and reciprocal behaviors that can be recognized.

In this case the ADHD son's (4) hyperactivity and school failure have been identified. By looking horizontally across his generation,

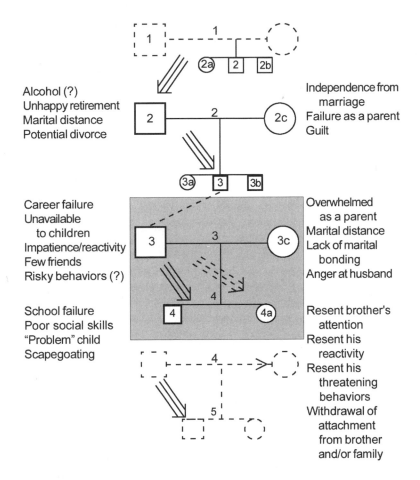

FIGURE 4.5. Primary and secondary ADHD symptoms in a five-generation family system.

within the sibling subsystem, we can speculate that his sister (4a) may be resentful of his "hyper" behaviors and the extra attention that he receives from his parents. She may feel left out of her parents' life and might develop her own behaviors to gain their attention and support. If she has even mild ADHD, inattentive type, symptoms, she will feel more alienated and unable to get her needs meet at home. If she struggles at school and socially, she will become more at risk for depression without receiving support from her parents. She may eventually distance herself from both her brother and her parents.

At the next generation level, the mother (3c) presents her own frustration and, perhaps, sense of failure as a parent due to her son's and daughter's behaviors. She may feel that she cannot effectively manage her ADHD son's life and that she has lost touch with her daughter. She may also feel anger and frustration with her husband since she gets little help from him with the children and feels that she is the sole caretaker. She may gradually distance herself emotionally from her husband. The father (3), whose ADHD is undiagnosed, may have internal problems of low self-esteem, a sense of failure from earlier school experiences, and uncertainty about the future of his career. He was probably the "problem child" or the "scapegoat" in his family of origin. If his disruptive behaviors caused conflict and resentment among his sisters (3a and 3b), he may have little contact with them as an adult. His impatience, temper, and emotional reactivity may have caused him problems at work as well as with his children and his marriage. He may have few friends, spend his time watching sports on television, and perhaps drink too much beer on the weekends.

Looking beyond the immediate nuclear family, it is also possible for the therapist to recognize other intergenerational patterns, as well as predisposing factors. The father (3), in his family of origin, may have experienced his own frustrations and perhaps failures at school as an undiagnosed ADHD child. His restless and hyperactive behaviors, in contrast to his better behaved sisters, could have made him a target for scapegoating. His own father's (2) potential ADHD may have created distance and impatience in the parent–child relationship (perhaps experienced by all three siblings). He may not be close to his sisters (3a and 3b) today as adults due to childhood conflicts and resentments. If his mother (2c) had played the role of "rescuer," positive memories of growing up may be primarily associated with his feelings of having been protected by her. His memories of his parents' styles of communication and interaction may be poor. He may view his own father, who is now approaching retirement age, as an unhappy and impatient man, often bickering with his wife, not involved with his marriage, and perhaps struggling with a drinking problem. These intergenerational patterns of ADHD symptoms and their circular and reciprocal interactions, while hypothetical, illustrate the underlying dynamics of family dysfunction. The recognition of these potentially dysfunctional intergenerational problems greatly enhances the therapist's resources for assessment and intervention. In recognizing the multilayering of clinical symptoms, based both on the ADHD and the resultant interactional patterns, the therapist can appreciate the need to continually work with the broader family dynamics. *These systemic influences are historically powerful for every family system and will overshadow the effectiveness of individual therapy for the ADHD child as well as the utility of stimulant medications.*

SYSTEMIC DYNAMICS IN ADHD FAMILY SYSTEMS

Intense and Persistent Vertical Loyalties

We have consistently observed in our practices that ADHD adults remain inordinately attached, in a continuing emotionally dependent manner, to their families of origin in general, and often to specific figures, such as a mother, a sibling, or a grandparent. This dependency is characterized by latent anger and unresolved emotional needs. We have not found any mention of this observation in the literature. Scapegoated children, while acting out their families' conflict, may remain emotionally tied to the family, which may provide a partial explanation of this dependency phenomenon. (For a discussion of the scapegoated child in the borderline family, see Everett et al., 1989; Everett & Volgy, 1998.)

This dependency factor is a component of what we have observed to be one of the more dramatic clinical patterns that occur in ADHD families: *an excessively high investment by the ADHD individual in intergenerational vertical loyalties.* Boszormenyi-Nagy and Spark (1973) described specific intergenerational patterns of bonding and attachment that occur between adults and their families of origin and with their spouses in terms of *family loyalties. Vertical loyalties* define an individual's emotional ties and continuing identities with their family of origin (see Figure 4.6). For example, developmentally, adolescents typically reduce these vertical ties to their parents and of family members as they approach young adulthood and begin to differentiate and seek more personal independence. As they prepare to leave home and separate from the family of origin, they further reduce these vertical ties so that they can develop more intimate personal relationships with adult peers.

Their new adult ties are described as horizontal loyalties. A task of

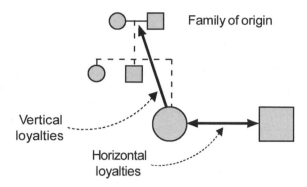

FIGURE 4.6. Vertical and horizontal loyalties in family systems.

all young adults in dating and mate selection is to *reduce their vertical ties and loyalties to their parents, and develop clear horizontal ties to their chosen partners.* Therapists recognize that this process creates early relationship problems for young adults in their first marriage where one, or both, partners are not clearly separated and differentiated from their families of origin. These vertical loyalties may continue to bind the individual such that these ties interfere with her or his availability to bond, and therefore develop horizontal loyalties, with their new partner.

Vertical and horizontal loyalties are powerful clinical dynamics that define clear "obligations" present, to varying degrees, for all family members. Examples can take numerous forms in family experiences:

> A 35-year-old wife may be called upon by the family to "take in" her younger brother when his marriage fails and he needs a place to live after completing a drug rehabilitation program.
> A 40-year-old husband may feel compelled to take out a second mortgage on his home in order to loan his parents $5,000 when his father's company closes unexpectedly.
> A married couple in their 50s may be expected to "take in" an aging parent after the other parent has died.

These loyalty issues can create clear dysfunctional patterns when vertical loyalties remain so powerful into adulthood that they interfere with and compromise the adult's marital relationship and other personal activities. The strength of these vertical loyalties is demonstrated, symbolically, in the frequency of contact between the adult and her or his family-of-origin members. For example, a husband may call his parents three or four times a week, even though their health is fine, and indicate that he "just needs to visit and chat."

We have observed that most ADHD adults carry internal scars, shadows of their childhood experiences with ADHD, arising from both home and school experiences. The inattentive child's negative experiences may have been relatively mild in terms of damage to self-esteem and self-confidence. However, the hyperactive child typically carries more serious negative self-images, deriving both from having been labeled "a problem child," "a screwup," "stupid," or "a failure" and from being scapegoated. These experiences seem to define the underlying dependency that we have just described. Just as injured birds stay close to their nests and wounded animals often return to their dens to die, the ADHD adult continually returns to the family "nest" or "den." Many ADHD children, and later adults, carry with them problematic threads of dependency that are tied to their families of origin. The more angry adults may overtly sever their emotional connection to their family of origin (as described by Bowen, 1978) by relocating thousands of miles away and restricting contact with their parents and/or siblings. However, they continue to live within the shadow of unanswered needs, and to suffer from unmet loyalties and obligations, hoping secretly, perhaps, that these will be resolved in the future.

These dynamics associated with the vertical loyalties of ADHD children and adults contribute to significant clinical patterns that require both family and individual clinical interventions. While not every ADHD family will display all of these systemic patterns, many will display some of them.

Poor Horizontal Loyalties in Marital Subsystems

Communication and interactive difficulties occur for ADHD adults in their marriages and other adult relationships. (These patterns will be discussed further in later chapters). Moreover, ADHD adults also experience difficulties bonding with their partners. The clinical and research literature has mistakenly assumed that the obvious marital difficulties present for ADHD couples are based solely on the detrimental influence of the ADHD symptoms, that is, restlessness, impulsivity, inattention, and distractibility. *But we have observed in many couples that the ADHD partner is often emotionally unavailable.* The spouse certainly identifies and complains about the ADHD symptoms and their impact on the relationship, but also admits something like "He is just not present," "I can't tell what's inside him," or "She never settles down to just be with me." Many ADHD adults apparently never prioritize their marital relationship by shifting their commitment from primarily vertical to primarily horizontal loyalties.

ADHD adults who have attempted to cut off their emotional ties with their families of origin also tend to do the same with their spouses and their children when stresses or unhappiness become problematic. Impulsivity and reactivity play a partial role in this dynamic. However, we have observed that many divorcing ADHD adults display a surprising ease in disconnecting and removing themselves from marriages, even long-term ones. We believe that divorce is so easy for these people—at least in part—because their horizontal loyalties to their spouses and children are weaker than their historical vertical loyalties to their families of origin.

Dysfunctional Patterns Occur in Enmeshing or Disengaging Systems

Family systems theory defines general interactive and emotional patterns of families in terms of an "enmeshing" or a "disengaging" process. *Enmeshing family systems* are highly interactive emotionally, such that feelings and events experienced by one member spread quickly through the family and are experienced by other members across the intergenerational system. However, some members may experience the intensity of this emotionality as problematic. If a child grows up in an enmeshing family system, he or she will benefit from the resource of handling emotional dynamics well, but he or she may also experience greater difficulty in separating from the family, leaving home, and creating his or her own autonomous identity. Highly enmeshing family systems are often described as *centripetally binding* (Stierlin, 1974, 1973), which means that the energy of the system serves to bind individual members' identifies and loyalties tightly to the family, which inhibits normal developmental separation.

Disengaging family systems are characterized by internal distance, fewer emotional ties, and fewer channels of interaction. Family members are often less aware of what is happening in the lives of other family members, even siblings and parents. The child who grows up in a disengaging family system is able to "leave home," separate, and individuate much more easily than the child in an enmeshing system. However, these individuals experience discomfort with intimacy and emotionality since both were lacking in their own family's interaction. They tend to avoid emotionally charged situations, and they struggle with partners who need closeness and availability. Highly disengaging family systems are often described as *centrifugal*, which means that the family tends to push members out of the system and away from further emotional connectedness (Stierlin, 1974, 1973).

Difficulties for ADHD children and adults appear to exist equally in enmeshing and in disengaging family systems. The patterns of vertical loyalties are somewhat stronger in enmeshing systems, but they are also present in disengaging systems. However, marital interactional patterns for ADHD adults vary somewhat because the non-ADHD spouse from an enmeshing family system expects greater emotional availability from her or his partner than does the spouse from a disengaging system.

Dependency and Immaturity Are Reinforced by Intergenerational Patterns

A family member's ADHD diminishes and deters successful family, social, and school adjustments, and creates additional problems of low self-esteem, low self-confidence, dependency, and immaturity. These issues exist in families as both symptoms of the ADHD member and, at the same time, as parental models for children. The ADHD child's personal and academic struggles engender both dependency on the family and immaturity. If a parent also has ADHD, her or his own dependency will become a model for the children through both parenting and marital interactions. The ADHD parent also displays her or his own immaturity through interactions and functions with her or his partner and children. These patterns are modeled and subsequently learned by all of the children, not just the ADHD child.

In families with an ADHD parent who has strong vertical loyalties with his or her family of origin, children will observe that parent's relative unavailability and reliance on his or her own parents. In some families a grandparent may be more emotionally available to a child than the ADHD parent. In other families grandparents may be distant and self-absorbed.

Low Self-Esteem and Personal Failure Are Reinforced by Interactive and Intergenerational Patterns

Many ADHD individuals experience a profound sense of failure, often expressed as feelings that they have never been "good enough" to please their parents, teachers, friends, and/or spouses. They often experience a sense of hopelessness about their future or their ability to be successful. Inadequacy often parallels these feelings. Many describe these feelings as a "shadow lurking inside," ready to emerge when frustrations or setbacks occur. Others describe the feeling as a "bottomless pit" of neediness and insecurity. Many ADHD individuals with these feelings display a constant need for reassurance and attention: children expect continuous reassurance from their parents, teachers, and even friends; adults expect these needs to be met by their spouses, parents, colleagues, and even their own children.

These patterns of low self-esteem arise from at least three sources:

1. Chronic behavioral and academic struggles and failures based on the ADHD disorder itself cause one to question one's abilities and self-worth.
2. Additional failures are reinforced interactively by scapegoating and the negative responses of frustrated parents, siblings, peers, and teachers.
3. Fewer resources are available in families that include an ADHD parent and/or grandparent, who experience his or her own sense of failure and low self-esteem because of an inability to meet the needs of the ADHD child.

The ADHD child's desire to please and to be loved is often met by anger and rejection, or simply unavailability, from her or his parents and siblings. These experiences engender an underlying sense of being *unlovable* as well as being incapable of *pleasing* the people on whom the ADHD child depends.

A Pervasive Sense of Guilt Often Exists across the Family Generations

One of the most interesting intergenerational patterns that we have observed in ADHD families is a sense of both personal and role-related guilt. In some families the guilt may be subtle, but in others it is overt. Adults often speak apologetically of their "failures" as parents with their ADHD child. These apologies may occur quite publicly, for example, during school conferences, even in front of their child, with teachers and school counselors. One father who was embarrassed that he was requested to attend such a meeting because of his son's failures and disruptive behaviors in school stated, "I apologize to each of you for John's behaviors. We did not raise our children to be like this." A mother who began to weep as she heard the teachers complain and describe her son's behaviors said, "I am so sorry that you have had to put up with this from Billy." Another mother, whose husband had recently divorced her for a younger woman after 18 years of marriage, reported that their last fight before the separation was prompted by their two ADHD sons' chronic problems. The husband had accused her of "never being able to handle these children." He felt that she had undermined his attempts to provide structure and discipline. She replied, "I am sorry that I protected them so much, I never wanted you to leave." (We will discuss the role of guilt in parental marital relationships, as well as the parental roles of "rescuer" and "disciplinarian," in Chapters 6 and 7).

Surprisingly both ADHD children and their siblings often express and share a similar sense of guilt. Many ADHD children, particularly the inattentive type, will often admit to their sadness for disappointing their parents and teachers and refer to themselves as "dumb," "stupid," or "retarded." Some are much more sensitive to their experience of failure than many therapists or school counselors realize because it has been reinforced over time by their parents' continual disappointment with them. ADHD children who display more hyperactive and impulsive behavioral problems readily talk about their own frustrations trying, unsuccessfully, to control themselves. For example, a 10-year-old boy, in a family session with his parents and sister, tried to explain that "sometimes I can't turn my motor off." Another child who had been labeled as a "discipline problem" said, "I don't know what comes over me. I want to stop myself from hitting other kids but when I get mad it's like a bomb goes off and I can't control myself. I feel really bad afterward."

The siblings of ADHD children are not very forgiving. Their reciprocal responses to the ADHD behaviors range from confrontation to withdrawal. Some siblings express privately that they "feel sorry" for their brother or sister. They commonly admit that they "feel bad" for their parents' frustrations and struggles with their ADHD sibling. Occasionally, as adults, these non-ADHD siblings look back and reflect that they wish they could have been more "tolerant" of or "sympathetic" toward their sibling. Ironically, many of these adult siblings may have ADHD children of their own.

Once in a while a recently diagnosed ADHD adult may reflect on her or his childhood and express both remorse and guilt regarding "what I must have put my parents through." An ADHD father apologized in a family therapy session to his wife and three children, stating, "I am sorry I did not get help for this sooner."

Family guilt is an expression of the sense of failure that is experienced and shared by all the family members. It is truly a systemic phenomenon and illustrates well the concepts of reciprocal and shared emotions. At one level the guilt represents the specific failures of a child or a parent; at another level, the guilt is a manifestation of an awareness of failure shared by all the family members. Many families feel that even when they tried to work together they could not make their problems go away. We have found that it is much easier for families to justify their struggles in raising a physically handicapped, autistic, or even schizophrenic child because the symptoms and problems presented are clearly distinguishable from most "normal" behaviors. ADHD, in contrast, occurs in "normal" children who simply cannot do many of the things that our own parents instructed us to do: *sit still at the table, don't fight with your sister, keep your room clean, don't talk back, get good grades, respect your teachers, always do your homework, pay attention in class, never get into fights, respect your elders, try to get along with everyone.*

Separation–Individuation Difficulties
Follow Successive Generations

The developmental goal of *separation–individuation* appears first any time from 18 months to approximately 3 years of age when a child's locomotion leads her or him to move physically away from the parents and test the safety of separateness. It occurs again when adolescents attempt to attain an identity apart from their parents and family. It is asserted finally when the young adult leaves home to live independently and eventually to marry.

For most ADHD adolescents and young adults this natural progression toward separation and individuation is inhibited and flawed. Some ADHD adolescents remain so immature and dependent on their families that they fall far behind their peers in achieving separation–individuation. Their experience of failures and conflicts at home, in school, and with their peers inhibit their ability and desire to look ahead to a life independent of their families. When the therapist asks "What do you think about doing when you finish high school?," the response may be a blank stare. Most do not plan ahead for even everyday tasks, so it is not surprising that they cannot think in terms of long-term tasks, let alone their own future.

ADHD adolescents tend to experience life solely in the present and indicate little interest in the future. One of the authors (CAE), who works with many ADHD adolescents, often interrupts a session by going to his waiting room to find a travel magazine. He brings it back and then asks the adolescent to look at the pictures and find scenes of places that look interesting enough to visit. Usually this exercise elicits little response from the adolescent. Sometimes he asks the adolescent to take the magazine home and mark the pages displaying locations that she or he might like to visit, or he suggests that the adolescent ask her or his parents what exciting places they have visited in the past. Occasionally these exercises help the adolescent begin to look beyond the present. However, for the

ADHD adolescent struggling to survive in school, the future is antici-
pated as a time as painful as the present. Sometimes, however, the therapist can work with a creative school counselor to help stimulate a high
school student's interest in college and to aid him or her in defining
future career issues. Unfortunately, for many ADHD adolescents, pro-
longed dependency will follow them into their young adult lives and
impact their choices of mates and careers.

CLINICAL MARKERS IN THE INTERGENERATIONAL TRANSMISSION OF ADHD

The clinician must be able to recognize significant clinical markers and
patterns that are present at varying levels for most ADHD families.
The therapist needs to recognize other influences, beyond the presenting symptoms, that are present in the life experiences of the ADHD
child or adult. The assessment and treatment process will be enhanced
by the therapist's awareness of these "markers."

The Bioneurological Condition

Research clearly supports the genetic factor in both the etiology and
the transmission of ADHD throughout the intergenerational family
system. The clinician must keep in mind the complexity of doing therapy with this disorder because it is composed of both biological and
emotional components. It is also a disorder that despite effective therapy and medication simply "will not go away." These resources provide, sometimes in dramatic fashion, the ADHD patient and her or his
family with a sense of control over, management of, and even accom-
plishment in overcoming ADHD symptoms, but they cannot "cure"
the underlying condition.

The clinician needs to understand this reality and be prepared to
discuss and explain it to patients and family members. The therapist's
ability to explicate these issues becomes critical at the onset of therapy
because of the tendency of parents, teachers, principals, and others to
try to "explain away" the disorder. Parents say to us, "He just needs to
grow up some more," or "If he were in different classes he would do
better," or "We can send him to live with my brother who was a
Marine—he'll straighten him out!" Tearful children or adolescents,
upon learning of their disorder, say to us or their parents, "Don't make
me take medicine, I'll try harder." While some of the symptoms are
more prominent at different ages and in differing contexts, their
minimalization, particularly after medical and/or therapeutic inter-

ventions, can cause many parents and teachers to believe that the disorder has been "cured" or is indeed "gone."

The most important early role for the therapist is to help families understand that ADHD is a clear disorder and then to *accept* its lifelong biological and emotional components. We feel badly for the ADHD child whose parents tell us, "We appreciate your help and concern, but we think Billy is just lazy. He doesn't need medication. We can manage this by being tougher and making him work harder." (We will discuss the family's response to medication issues in Chapter 6.)

Vertical Loyalties and Dependency

ADHD individuals tend to display a high incidence of binding vertical loyalties. Their personal and developmental struggles create patterns of emotional dependency on parents and their families of origin. This emotional binding represents, for both parents and the patients, a sense of safety and security despite the persistence of the struggles. These patterns may delay the adolescent's or young adult's separation–individuation and restrict his or her potential to establish firm horizontal loyalties in peer and sexual relationships.

In families with an ADHD parent, these patterns are exacerbated. An ADHD adult who exhibits excessive dependency may become attached to her or his spouse in such a way that he or she expects, even demands, to be "taken care of," and this expectation can easily lead to marital conflict.

Intergenerational Scapegoating

The role of the "family scapegoat," as we have discussed, has been recognized since the earliest works in family systems theory (Ackerman, 1958; Bell & Vogel, 1961). It is important to recognize that, while a child is assigned the role of scapegoat in the family, she or he also performs the role in school, peer group, and occupational settings. *The disruptive behaviors of the ADHD child, particularly the hyperactive–impulsive type, in these settings makes her or him an easy target for continued scapegoating.* The experience of the role is pervasive for the child because it is reinforced by parents, siblings, grandparents, aunts, uncles, cousins, teachers, principals, counselors, and peers. It is not hard to imagine, since there is little chance of escape from the role, why so many ADHD children and adolescents display symptoms of depression, anxiety, and/or oppositional behaviors.

Patterns of Emotional and Physical Abuse

The risk of abuse being displayed by ADHD, hyperactive–impulsive type, children, adolescents, and adults is supported in the literature. For children, this takes the form of bossiness or cruelty toward siblings, peers, parents, and even animals. Occasionally it can be magnified into physical violence toward parents or other adults. Frustrated and angry ADHD adolescents, who see themselves as failures at home, academically, and socially, are prone to displays of abuse and violence. For ADHD adults, the abuse behaviors may range from impatience and hypercriticalness toward spouses and children to outright aggression and violence. The ADHD components of impulsivity, reactivity, and intensity further dramatize the potential for abusive behaviors.

The lack of "self-regulation" for ADHD individuals is addressed in recent literature (Barkley, 1997), which notes that most ADHD individuals lack the ability to "inhibit" inappropriate behavior and that this inability derives from biological components. This lack of inhibition, Barkley suggests (1997), may be at the root of many dysfunctions seen in the behaviors of ADHD individuals.

The potential for violence by the ADHD adult, who carries lifelong frustrations into her or his adult relationships, is high. It is further heightened if the adult was subjected to abusive conditions by his or her own parents as a child. These behaviors for adults appear to be triggered primarily by stresses and conflicts in three settings: (1) the marriage, (2) parenting, and (3) work. Many intense and restless ADHD fathers tell us that they avoid playing with their young children because of their high levels of frustration. Others tell us that they are cannot sit quietly and read to their children at bedtime because of their impatience. Many report stories of impulsively "striking out" at a child who asked "too many questions," who "wouldn't settle down," or who "splashed me with bathtub water." Spouses tell us of "having to walk on eggshells" when their ADHD partner is around, fearful that making the "wrong" comment will cause a reactive outburst. It is important for the therapist to recognize that in some ADHD families this potential for abuse and violence has marked several generations and remains uncomfortably near the surface.

The potential for the ADHD child or adolescent to become the victim of emotional or physical abuse is also high. Intensely hyperactive infants and young children may suffer physical reactions from parents whose management skills are poor and whose frustration tolerances are low. The risk for abuse increases many fold if there are other

ADHD children or an ADHD parent in the family. Many children and adolescents receive considerable emotional abuse from frustrated parents, teachers, siblings, and friends. We have observed that the weaker the parent's management skills, the greater will be the potential for abusive conditions, either emotionally or physically, in the family.

Persistent Models of Poor Parental Control and Interaction

The high levels of frustration experienced by parents of ADHD children, and their ongoing struggles to manage behaviors and academic problems, create poor management and structural outcomes and divert parents' attention and energy away from the other children in the family, as well as from their own personal needs and joint relationship. Parental struggles often dominate spouses' communication, interaction, and image of the family. (We will discuss the frustration and rejection experienced by siblings later in this chapter). Children who grow up in families in which there is a continuing struggle for control and stability by the parents do not experience effective models of parental management or interaction, and also feel left out of family interaction.

The ADHD parent (as well as her or his adult siblings) has typically learned inadequate models of parenting and management from their own family of origin. Most of these adults reenact, in their own nuclear families, the ineffective models that they experienced and witnessed. Such models were even more inadequate where an ADHD parent was present.

Persistent Models of Inadequate and/or Reactive Parenting

Frustrated parents of ADHD children report their own continuing sense of inadequacy and feelings that they are ineffective in their parenting skills and roles. Typically they lack consistency, firmness, and structure, as well as an ability to confer and function as a coparent team with their spouse. This sense of inadequacy leads many parents to engage in reactive, if not abusive, responses toward their children. The scapegoated ADHD child is not the only recipient of this frustration, which spills over toward other children, the spouse, or even colleagues in the work setting. *Non-ADHD siblings often describe their parents as unpredictable, reactive, harsh, punitive, uncaring, disinterested, and mean.* Even in less reactive parental situations, the ADHD child often does not understand why his or her parents need to be firmer and more consistent with him or her, while the nonADHD siblings wonder why their parents do not enforce limits and discipline consistently for their ADHD sibling.

When ADHD has been present over several generations, the parental models in the ADHD families of origin are marred by similar degrees of frustration, inadequacy, and reactivity. These models are transmitted not only to the ADHD child, but to the siblings, who also go on to carry these models into their own adult parenting roles.

Persistent Models of Sibling Conflict and/or Rejection

Non-ADHD siblings provide important windows into the frustrations, and often chaos, present in the clinical family system. The therapist must regard these siblings as resources and involve them in both the assessment and treatment processes. They are rarely at a loss for words in criticizing their ADHD sibling and their parents. Many have been in physical confrontations with their sibling, while others report feeling intimidated or abused by the sibling. In addition to the anger and frustration they feel, most will communicate a sense of "rejection" that they experience as the result of their parents' preoccupation and struggles with the ADHD sibling. This feeling is particularly apparent in families where the ADHD child is hyperactive and impulsive.

In one single-parent family, the 16-year-old adolescent boy was relied upon by his working mother to help manage and control his 9-year-old hyperactive ADHD brother. Their 13-year-old sister kept to herself and had already distanced from the ADHD brother. The 16-year-old was often asked to be in charge of the home while the mother was at work or out with friends, which gave him a sense of status (he had been parentified) in the household due to the absence of his father. (This is a pattern seen in many single-parent family systems.) However, his role often triggered resentment and reactivity in the younger ADHD brother, who responded by breaking household items and kicking holes in the wall. The older brother became increasingly physical in his attempts to control his brother.

One night, while the mother was out, the two engaged in a confrontation after the older brother had tried to make the sibling pick up his clothing. The ADHD child threw a shoe and shattered a large window. The brother grabbed the 9-year-old, trying to restrain him and carry him to his bedroom. The more the sibling resisted, the more physical the brother became, until the confrontation resulted in bloody noses and bruises. When the mother arrived home, she reacted immediately to the violence by blaming the 16-year-old, not the ADHD child. He responded by blaming her. She called the police, fearing that he was "out of control." By the time they arrived everyone had calmed down, but, since there were physical injuries to the younger son, the brother was arrested and spent the night in juvenile detention.

The situation just described, while dramatic, is not unusual in ADHD families. It can also occur in families where one parent, usually the father, travels frequently or is simply uninvolved in the parenting. These non-ADHD older siblings who are expected to perform parentified roles often feel resentful about their roles. Many will leave the home abruptly and prematurely (as did the older brother in the above case, who moved across the country to live with his biological father). The overall sibling relationships in many of these ADHD families are often so damaged that the effects will carry over into their adult years.

Persistent Attitudes for Educational Failure

Clear attitudes regarding educational failure are often present throughout ADHD families. Where one or both parents are high achievers, the sense of educational failure is further dramatized in the struggles of their ADHD child. When there is an ADHD parent, or even an ADHD grandparent, in the family, these attitudes may be reinforced by years of academic and occupational difficulties. The father who struggled with undiagnosed ADHD in school, who never felt that he was able to achieve the success he or his parents expected, may communicate a disdain for education to his children. He might make excuses for the disruptive behaviors of his ADHD child and blame the child's problems on the teacher (which he learned to do as a child). He defends his child by stating, "That's not a big deal, I did all of that myself."

Such lack of support for educational attainment creates conflicts with spouses who want their children to be successful. It also can create severe conflict with grandparents. For example, in this case, the paternal grandparents may side with the ADHD father, who is not pushing the child, since they struggled with the father's (their son's) own upbringing and educational failures; the maternal grandparents may side with the mother in upholding higher achievement standards for the child and investing for the grandchild's college education.

These patterns lead to considerable inconsistency by the parents in their management of school difficulties for their ADHD child (and often their other children). This creates significant emotional and self-identify problems for the ADHD child and severely inhibits her or his outlook on schooling.

Persistent Poor Modeling for Social Skills and Personal Decision Making

Many ADHD individuals—whether children or adults—display poor social skills and impaired social judgments. It is difficult for ADHD individuals to accurately perceive and recognize other persons' potential responses or reactions in social situations. They often lack sufficient empathy to judge the potential impact of their behaviors in interactional situations. The ADHD child and adolescent often lack peer friends because her or his behaviors have offended or irritated them. Other peers may experience the ADHD child as socially inept or immature. Their social skills may lag 2 or more years behind those of their peers. The ADHD adult is similarly lacking in these same skills, which diminishes his or her social network and causes him or her to rely solely on a spouse to arrange and support social activities for them.

Even socially successful parents may offer inadequate modeling for their children due to their ongoing stress and management struggles. In families with an ADHD parent, social skills models are even more limited. Many spouses of ADHD partners report that their partners' behaviors are "like having another child in the family." The ADHD parent often displays a lack of sensitivity and empathy within the family relationships. This model can become more problematic when children observe the ADHD parent's negative reactives, demeaning remarks, chronic criticisms, or confrontational behaviors. These sabotage the potentially good modeling offered by the non-ADHD parent.

Persistent Low Self-Worth

The life experiences of ADHD individuals often carry the painful threads of chronic low self-esteem and low self-worth. Their histories are often colored by their senses of failure and ineptness. These perceptions are reinforced further by the often angry and rejecting interactions they have experienced since childhood with parents, siblings, peers, and teachers. The persistence of this negative feedback is internalized as a seriously devalued sense of self. Few ADHD children or adults can state that they have experienced more positive feedback than negative feedback over their lifetimes. It does not take long for the child to internalize the message that she or he is a failure and worthless.

The ADHD individual's development is characterized by the beliefs that "anything I try will fail" and "I will never satisfy Mom and Dad." Many eventually decide that it is better not to try at all than to risk failure and ridicule again. These negative experiences for the ADHD child cast a persistent and lifelong shadow over her or his self-image and self-confidence. They begin to select peers with similarly low self-esteem and poor levels of personal and academic achievement. As one bright ADHD adolescent said, "I hang out with the nonconformists in high school because they are the only ones I feel comfortable with and can talk to."

This sense of personal despair begins for many ADHD children as early as fifth or sixth grade and can turn into angry acting-out behaviors. Soon these ADHD children are labeled oppositional defiant. Much like a child who has been physically or sexually abused, many young ADHD adolescents can identify their inner sense of rage. However, the ADHD adolescent cannot pinpoint the causes of these feelings and talk openly about feeling oppressed, rejected, or "getting even."

Persistent Models of Marital Conflict

Marital dissatisfaction and conflict is persistent and underlies most relationships in which an ADHD child or partner (or both) is present. This conflict exist on a variety of personal and interactive levels (this topic will be discussed further in Chapter 8). As we have indicated, the stresses of parental management simply "spill over" and intrude into the marriage. Many spouses report that most of their personal interaction and communication, even when they are out alone together at a movie or having dinner privately, is dominated by the problems of their ADHD child and/or other children. They have difficulty making private time for one another. The chronicity of this parental difficulties eventually damages the quality of their marital interaction and eventually their mutual bonding and trust.

When one of the spouses is also ADHD, the marital problems are even more pronounced. The adult symptoms, in addition to the parental management issues, create another layer of problems that disrupt both parental dialogue and marital interaction. These marriages are often characterized by poor communication, limited privacy and intimacy, poor coparenting and problem solving, deteriorating bonding and trust, and emotional reactivity and potential violence.

These 11 clinical markers are intended to highlight for the clinician the broader systemic patterns that are often present and that characterize dysfunctional interactions in addition to the member's ADHD symptoms. They describe the broader clinical dimensions of a family system's response to the presence of the ADHD disorder. We will expand discussion of all these issues in the following clinical chapters.

5

A Five-Stage Developmental Model for Assessing ADHD throughout the Family System

The role of assessment and diagnosis is central to clinical work with ADHD individuals and their families. Regarding the broader family system, an accurate assessment involves acquiring an understanding of the family's structure and history; the ADHD individual's behavioral, educational, and social history; parent and teacher observations; psychometric assessment of cognitive functioning; consideration of differential diagnoses; and the clinician's observations. Since ADHD is basically a bioneurological disorder, its presence (diagnosed or not) is lifelong, with continuing serious ramifications for these children and their families. In addition, ADHD individuals are often at high risk for comorbid psychiatric disorders that may actually camouflage the ADHD symptoms.

In this chapter we will identify the ADHD symptoms as they appear in five developmental life stages:

1. The infant and toddler years.
2. The preschool and kindergarten years.
3. The early grade school years.
4. The later grade school years.
5. The middle and high school years.

Within each of these stages we will identify the symptomatic patterns as they occur throughout the family system:

1. For the symptomatic individual.
2. For the parent–child subsystem.
3. For the sibling subsystem.
4. For the marital subsystem.

A developmental model provides therapists with a clinical frame of reference, as well as a time line along which the complex clusters of ADHD symptoms can be tracked for the identified individual in the context of the family system. Furthermore, it provides a conceptual orientation for developing specific treatment strategies and interventions at differing stages in the family's life cycle.

The clinician's ability to recognize ADHD symptoms and the family's reciprocal responses enhance the potential for accurate diagnosis and appropriate treatment planning. Since the formal diagnosis of ADHD relies heavily on reports of early symptoms, the clinician evaluating an older child, adolescent, or adult will often need to question parents regarding the individual's behaviors as a young child. To interpret this information accurately, the clinician needs to understand how ADHD symptoms manifest in children of different ages, as well as how these symptoms are perceived and responded to by parents (We will use the plural for parents throughout our text for simplicity's sake, though we acknowledge the presence of single-parent ADHD families). For example, the mother of a hyperactive 12-year-old may report that she remembers her son as an infant being difficult to hold and often unresponsive to her, or that she remembers him being unusually sensitive to noise or touch. These early symptoms of ADHD in the infant, based on the mother's recall, are quite different from the present ADHD symptoms of the 12-year-old that the mother, teacher, and child report to the therapist now.

By placing these clinical observations in the context of family life-cycle stages, the clinician can track the effects of the disorder at any developmental level. Difficult behaviors that characterized the very young child can now be recognized as red flags that clinically support the diagnostic process. The cluster of ADHD symptoms (as well as the family's responses to them) will vary considerably across the life cycle, manifesting differently in a 5-year-old child, a 16-year-old adolescent, and a 35-year-old adult. The clinician's ability to recognize these differing symptoms and patterns, both in the ADHD individual and within his or her family's interactional dynamics, can speed early detection of the disorder and facilitate a more accurate clinical diagnosis. For example, a mother's response to learning that her first-grader has trouble sitting still in class and exhibits difficulty focusing on tasks will be quite different from the response of a mother who has been struggling for 8 years with similarly disruptive behaviors, school failure, and conduct disorder symptoms in her 14-year-old child.

After making the initial assessment the therapist creates a developmental profile to position the presenting problematic behaviors in the context of the individual's immediate and historical life setting and provide a broader view of family dynamics and responses. The greater the therapist's awareness of these dynamics within the ADHD family, the greater the therapist's opportunity to plan more thoughtful and clinically relevant therapeutic strategies and interventions. For example, the clinician working with a grade school-age ADHD child must make routine clinical choices about how often and in what setting (i.e., interview or play) to work with the child directly, how often to see the child's parents, when to see the child with the parents, and whether or when to involve siblings in the therapy process. The developmental profile will help the therapist answer these strategic clinical questions.

Our five-stage developmental model, which has evolved over the years of our clinical experiences with ADHD families, initially identifies the child's specific ADHD symptoms as they appear in their respective life-cycle stages: for example, the patterns as they appear in infancy as compared to patterns in early grade school or middle school. Next the model identifies the reciprocal interactive patterns within the family system of the parental and sibling responses to the child's ADHD symptoms. Finally, the model notes the effects of the ADHD symptoms on the parental marital relationship across these five stages. ADHD produces a ripple effect in a family, much like a pebble that is thrown into a pond of water. With our developmental model, we are able to track this ripple effect of ADHD symptoms throughout the reciprocal interactional patterns of the family system (see Table 5.1).

There will be exceptions to this model, of course. Every family is unique, and thus a family's responses to the ADHD symptoms may differ somewhat from our"typical" model at one stage or another. Certain parental or marital responses may begin at stages earlier or later than we have described, usually due to the severity of the child's symptoms and/or the absence of sufficient parenting resources. In addition, for the sake of better illustration and greater clarity, we have not tried to identify the more complex patterns wherein ADHD is present in two or more children in one family or shared by intergenerational family members, particularly parents. The complexity of these potential patterns and their intergenerational transmission have been illustrated in the genograms in Chapter 4. We will, however, allude to examples where both a child and a parent have been diagnosed with

TABLE 5.1. Five Life-Cycle Stages of a Family's Experience with an ADHD Child

Time period	The child's experience	Parental response	Sibling response	Marital response
Stage 1: Infant and toddler years	Bioneurological etiology	"Different" and/or "damaged" child Inadequate bonding Struggle with acceptance Denial	Awareness of "differentness" of ADHD sibling	Increased stress Blaming one another
Stage 2: Preschool and kindergarten years	Inattentiveness Distractibility Impulsivity Hyperactivity Parental disputes	Excessive time demands Management problems Feelings of inadequacy and frustration Reduced time with other children	Early sibling conflicts Rivalry and jealousy Reduced time from parent	Communication and intimacy inhibited by parental stress Reduced private time Diffuse marital boundaries
Stage 3: Early grade school years	Emerging ego problems Self-management difficulties Learning frustrations and/or delays Impaired social skills	Discouragement and hopelessness Ambivalence for giving love and nurturance Increased management problems "Critical" and "Protector" parental roles emerge	Anger and argumentativeness Rejection and isolation of sibling	Diminished communication and intimacy Heightened stress Mutual withdrawal of emotional support
Stage 4: Later grade school years	Conduct difficulties at home and/or school Comorbid symptoms of anxiety, depression, and/or oppositional behaviors Increasing educational problems	Anger and punitiveness Scapegoating of ADHD child and potential for abuse Feelings of helplessness and inadequacy with ADHD child	Alienation and withdrawal of affect from ADHD sibling and family Physical confrontations with ADHD sibling	Conflicts intensified and generalized from parental arena to everyday interactions Increased distancing and deterioration of communication
Stage 5: Middle and high school years	General problematic behaviors School failure, truancy, and dropping out Substance abuse Reactivity to parents Conflicts in the community Aborted attempts to run away from home	External pressures from school, community, courts, etc. Embarrassment in community and intergenerational family Sense of parental failure Continued scapegoating Heightened abuse potential Withdrawal of nurturance	Acting-out behaviors and/or emotional reactivity Physical withdrawal from the family	Marital failure Depression Alienation from one another Potential for separation and/or divorce

ADHD. Therapists should be able to extrapolate the added levels of stress, frustration, and crisis throughout a family system where additional members display ADHD symptoms.

While it is evident that the clinical patterns identified throughout this model will be present in most families whether or not a formal ADHD diagnosis has been made, therapists should recognize that the actual diagnosis may occur at many locations across this model. Often the earliest red flags signaling the possible presence of ADHD do not come from the symptomatic individual, who may have been referred for any number of comorbid conditions, but from the comments, reflections, and experiences reported by parents or spouses (in the case of adults). Therefore, it is important for the clinician to be able to recognize the cluster of symptomatic ADHD behaviors as they manifest in the various life-cycle stages *and* as they are experienced and reported by other family members, *even when there has not been a consideration of ADHD by the family or the therapist.* Of course, the earlier the symptoms are recognized and the child (or adult) diagnosed, the more effective the interventions can be and the more successful parents, teachers, and therapists can be in preventing and/or correcting emotional damage.

STAGE 1: THE INFANT AND TODDLER YEARS

There is a distinct clinical advantage with regard to treatment outcomes when a child is diagnosed with ADHD in the preschool years, or even in the first few years of grade school. Unfortunately, most parents have great difficulty dealing with and accepting such an early diagnosis. Children who are diagnosed at this early age are predominantly hyperactive–impulsive types. Parents of these children can articulate clearly that their young child has "always been difficult" or "is not like my other children," and often lament, "I have read every parenting book available to try to understand what I can do, and nothing has worked." By comparison, the ADHD inattentive child may not be recognized and diagnosed until the end of grade school or even into middle or high school.

The Young Child's Experience

The young child's most prominent symptoms are typically hyperactive in nature and include the inability to sit still, constant squirming and fidgeting, sometimes wild risk-taking in play, and often a reluctance to be held or cuddled. This may be a child who, during his or her first year of life, *never* slept through an entire night. ADHD babies are marked by a high incidence of colic, and occasionally by food allergies and/or eating difficulties. They may refuse to suckle long enough to breast-feed successfully. Breast-feeding is therefore terminated prematurely, thus leaving the mother with an early sense of parenting failure. These infants often display extreme tactile and auditory sensitivities. Some may cry incessantly because their sheets are too stiff, their clothing too hot, or their garments too constraining. Others may be overly sensitive in their reaction to loud or sudden noises in their environment. Some ADHD infants cry all the time and are unwilling to be consoled. Some ADHD toddlers actually walk before they crawl. They appear to be fearless, often exploring their environment earlier, more eagerly, and without typical levels of caution.

These young children may also have difficulties with toilet training; males often remain untrained until very late. They may have soiling problems because they do not take the time to wipe themselves properly. They can be quite resistant to taking time away from their play activities to go to the bathroom. Thus they often have "accidents" because they wait too long, and this can be frustrating to their parents, who then must help with the cleanup. The more hyperactive children can be difficult to take anywhere outside of the home in these early years because they are so difficult to control. Parents often feel great pressure trying to keep the child adequately occupied or managed. Eating out at restaurants or even going to the grocery store can be frustrating and exhausting experiences. Consequently, many parents begin very early to curtail their outings together, so that one parent can stay home with the ADHD child while the other takes care of errands and other social needs.

Typically, these young children are easily distracted and emotionally reactive. Many will have great difficulty delaying gratification and handling frustration. Thus, not only do necessary trips to the store become difficult, but "fun" trips to zoos or amusement parks or any other places where standing in line, waiting one's turn, or paying attention to dangers is necessary can be a very trying experience for their parents. When parents attempt to manage the child's behaviors in these settings, the child may create loud and embarrassing scenes in public. Other family members' attempts to enjoy the occasion are often spoiled.

The parents of three children, the youngest of whom was a hyperactive 5-year-old, reported that their two older children were angry at them because they had suspended all family activities the prior year. They had endured episodes of the ADHD child "running wild" through movie theaters and "disappear-

ing" in shopping malls. In the latter situation the older brother found the child "playing" inside a large dumpster behind the mall stores. He was discovered only after the frantic family and mall security had been searching for him for nearly 1 hour. The "final straw" came when the family was having dinner at a busy fast-food restaurant. The ADHD child had gone to the bathroom but instead of returning to the table he ventured out into the parking lot. The family was alerted by the sound of car horns blaring from the parking lot. When they ran outside, they found the missing child standing on the rear bumper of a delivery truck that was pulling out of the lot—the driver was unaware of the child's presence.

The Parental Response

It is painfully apparent that a couple's joyous expectations of parenthood can be easily crushed with the advent of an ADHD child. The expected infant, the one who coos and cuddles and listens well and is actually fun to take places, is never experienced. Instead, the baby or emerging toddler is an energetic dynamo who "won't sleep," "won't eat," "cries easily," has colic for long periods of time, is "willful and demanding," and often hates to be cuddled. Parents of such a child naturally feel despondent, discouraged, angry, and confused. In their hearts they want to be the best parents possible, but they find themselves instead yelling and spanking and, at times, feeling hateful toward this child whom they also love desperately. They begin to feel that they have been dealt a "raw deal" and that this parenting experience is "unfair." They may feel frightened by the volatility of their own emotions and be afraid or ashamed to express them honestly, even to one another. They doggedly begin the long process of trying to make sense of what seems to them nonsensical: "How can this child not respond lovingly to my loving parenting?" "What did we do wrong?"

We worked with one mother who cried during most of her sessions due to her sense of guilt and failure because she was unable to enjoy her 5-year-old son. She finally confessed that she feared that she "secretly hated" her son and often "wished that I had never had him" because he had made her life "a living hell." The mother's despondency was great and her guilt often overwhelming. As she worked on these feelings in therapy, it became clear to us that the most painful issue for her was that her son, who was her first, had been desired for a very long time and his conception had been planned. Her images of motherhood, which had included having a "sweet baby" and enjoying the closeness of being a devoted mother, were shattered by the daily reality of parenting this hyperactive ADHD child. The mother was depressed and grieving over the lost fantasy of the motherhood that "should have been."

In frustration, parents may turn on one another in accusation and blame: "What are *you* doing wrong?" "Why can't *you* manage him better?" Unfortunately, their attempts to find answers to these questions often take place in a void, without the support and information they need from their pediatricians or family physicians, who are the "authorities" they most often turn to for help. Too often pediatricians dismiss these early worries and fears as "new parent's anxiety" and fail to give thoughtful consideration to the presentation of symptoms that might indicate ADHD. Ironically, they may even point out the advantages of having a child with high activity levels, praising the problem child as "high-spirited" or "all boy." They may also tell the parents that they need to relax and "enjoy the experience," thus contributing to their sense of incompetency and guilt.

The undiagnosed ADHD child will often be labeled by parents as *different* or *difficult*. If he or she is not their first child, they will lament over how different this one is from the others. They will wonder why their newest child is not more "cuddly" or does not allow them to "do things for her [him]" like they had been able to do with their older children. Some parents begin to look for medical reasons for the child's problem behaviors or try an endless and futile series of practical interventions, like changing the child's diet or becoming more restrictive. Other parents try to impose new behavior, such as forcibly cuddling the young child in the hope that she or he will relax and begin to "like it" after a while. Of course, this strategy often leads to dramatic tantrums and the child's even greater resistance to the parent. If this is their first child, they will often comment, "This is never what I expected being a mom was going to be like" or "My mother never told me it would be this difficult."

When the child is diagnosed accurately at some point during these early years, it often confirms the parents' belief or fear: "I knew something was wrong." But for many young parents an early diagnosis of ADHD prompts a profound sadness, tears, even a sense of hopelessness. Even when we explain the diagnosis to them, they respond as if we had told them that their child was dying of leukemia. Many parents translate their reactive emotions into the perception that their child is "damaged." They may even turn their disappointment into anger and blame directed at their spouse by saying something like "I always knew there was something wrong with your mother," or "Your family has always been weird—I should have never married you," or even "I always told you that we should not have smoked all that dope during college."

For some, the diagnosis is met with strong denial. We try to encourage these parents to read more about ADHD and to consult with some of our educational and medical colleagues. In an effort to help them accept and understand both the diagnosis and their own fears, we may ask them to talk to our educational consultant to gain some assurance that most ADHD children who are treated appropriately do fine in school. It may take several months or longer before some parents can accept the diagnosis and see a future for their child and a direction for treatment. As in other general grief experiences, there is considerable blaming of self and/or other. Often parents will spend many sessions talking about their sense of inadequacy in parenting, reiterating the fear that "I must have done something wrong" and the hope that "there must be a simpler solution."

The Sibling Response

Older siblings of very young ADHD children tend not to be as reactive to or competitive with the ADHD child at this early stage as they can become with a later-stage ADHD sibling. They will often describe their ADHD sibling as "weird" or "different," "a pain" or "a brat." Sometimes they will wonder why their parents do not discipline or control the ADHD sibling more or better. It is common for an older child to give her or his parents advice about how to handle the troublesome sibling and even take on the role of an assistant parent. Sometimes this response occurs because the parents have actively enlisted the aid of the older child to help with monitoring the ADHD child, since such a child requires a great deal more supervision. Sometimes this older sibling may see that her or his parents are frustrated and angry and may voluntarily take on an assistant parenting role to try to help them feel better. When an older sibling is allowed or encouraged to take on this "parentified" role, this is a sign that the family's patterns of adaptation are becoming dysfunctional.

Younger non-ADHD siblings may show their frustration through more regressive behaviors. Since their ADHD sibling requires so much of their parents' energy and attention, they may become more dependent in order to compete for the attention they need; for example, they may shadow their parents and want to be with them all the time. They may also exhibit anger, stubbornness, or oppositional behaviors directed at their parents for not paying them the same amount of attention that they perceive their ADHD sibling receives.

In some families, especially when the child has not yet been diagnosed with ADHD, the non-ADHD siblings will tell us that they feel embarrassed or shamed by the way their ADHD sibling behaves. They may regard their sibling as different, shunning or demeaning her or him in front of friends. The diagnosis of ADHD often brings a sense of relief to the entire family. However, family members they may also feel guilty about the shame they felt and about how they treated their ADHD sibling before the problem was identified.

The Marital Response

Typically, parents of young children are young adults who have been away from their own families of origin for only a couple of years. Probably married only a few years, they may still be seeking closure to their own developmental process of family separation and working to establish an adult intimate relationship. The earliest challenge to their new relationship is understanding how to become parents in the context of defining and protecting their marital intimacy and establishing boundaries with their families of origin. For most young couples, the experience of pregnancy and the presence of an infant is a mixed blessing, requiring many adjustments in their former lifestyle. The intrusion of an ADHD child, particularly when hyperactive, into a young marriage can cause serious disruption of and sometimes permanent damage to the relationship.

Experiencing adjustments to new parenthood *and* the high stress associated with an ADHD child can permeate the couple's early relationship and eventually affect their everyday interactions on all levels, from verbal communication to sexual intimacy. Increasingly serious marital conflicts follow, which may include disillusionment, anger, and distance. Partners frequently find themselves in conflict over parenting strategies and begin to blame one another for their ineffectiveness and/or frustration. Their own inexperience and lack of maturity may also contribute to difficulty managing their feelings of anger and frustration with the child. In some young families this can lead to an early potential for abuse, either toward the child or in the marriage. These early conflicts will continue to develop and accumulate over time and can be recognized by the therapist whether or not a child has already been diagnosed with ADHD.

STAGE 2: THE PRESCHOOL
AND KINDERGARTEN YEARS

The ADHD child who is diagnosed in these early years typically shows symptoms of impulsivity, hyperactivity, and distractibility. The symptoms of ADHD children who are predominantly inattentive in nature are often not recognized by parents or teachers at this early age; indeed, for these primarily inattentive children, particularly those who are intellectually above average, the ADHD symptoms may not be recognized until late grade school or early middle school. The more impulsive ADHD child entering kindergarten or first grade has experienced several years of being corrected or admonished by parents: "Slow down," "Learn to control yourself," "Don't get into that," "Why can't you listen to what I tell you?" These common symptoms representing the early cluster of ADHD behaviors are typically stated quite clearly in the parents' report of their child's early years.

The Child's Experience

Many young ADHD children are placed in daycare or preschool at fairly young ages because the primary caregiving parent needs a break. If they are in daycare, they may already have a history of experiencing difficulty getting along with other children, and being criticized, scolded, and put in time-out by other adult caregivers. In preschool, these are the children who cannot sit still during story time, will not settle down during nap times, and will not share their toys. They are noticeably more aggressive than other children; in fact, uncontrolled aggression is common among these young ADHD children because of the combination of impulsivity and volatility. They will often hit another child if he or she takes their toys away. Frequent temper tantrums over mildly upsetting events are an all-too-common pattern.

These behaviors pose difficulties for the preschool teacher because time-outs must be structured differently. The ADHD symptoms require that the child be more clearly separated or removed from classroom stimuli. Sadly, these children may begin to feel that others are united against them, that no one likes them, that everyone tries to get them in trouble, and that they cannot do anything right to please the adults around them. By the time many of these young ADHD children are entering first grade, signs of a poor self-image and lower self-esteem may already be present. Often they will be described by parents and caregivers as "unhappy" children who are difficult to please.

The Parental Response

Many parents of hyperactive–impulsive ADHD children (particularly mothers who have stayed at home during these early years) speak openly about their relief when their child is finally old enough to be in preschool. Freed from total responsibility for the child, they are often amazed to discover just how much energy and time they expended to care for the ADHD child as compared to their other children. However, some parents who were the child's primary caretaker and defender during these years may also assume even *more* parental responsibilities at this stage, often to the greater exclusion and neglect of other children. Some mothers spend several hours a day in the classroom with their child in order to monitor and manage her or his disruptive behaviors, "to save the child from being punished," and "to save the family from embarrassment." Some teachers and principals can tolerate this role and even develop it creatively, while others see it either as an intrusion into the normal functioning of the classroom or—worse—an "insult" to the teacher, who believes that she is better able to manage the ADHD child without the parent present. In fact, when we consult with these teachers about the child, we often learn that they view these mothers as overbearing and intrusive and try to find other duties to keep them out of their way.

Time demands on parents increase dramatically when their ADHD children are able to explore more and venture out into areas beyond their home surroundings. Keeping ADHD children occupied is important to both parents and teachers because they can be managed better when they are interested and involved in stimulating activities. However, active and exploring behaviors create further frustrations for parents who are attempting to monitor and supervise the ADHD child while keeping up with the needs of other children in the family. Disputes between parents often increase as parental time demands increase.

Other parents are simply relieved to send their ADHD child to school and would rather tolerate calls from teachers and principals. By the time their child enters school, these parents have already endured several years of parental frustration that has *demanded excessive time* and caused countless *behavioral management struggles*. The feedback given to these parents by teachers and other school personnel about their child's behaviors in school often makes their acceptance of the ADHD diagnosis at this stage somewhat easier, for their own frustrations are now finally confirmed. While denial is still sometimes present, it is much harder for parents at this stage to ignore the complaints of teachers when those complaints match what they have been telling themselves and their spouses for years.

These parents will readily voice their own continuing frustrations and their growing sense of inadequacy. These feelings of inadequacy are typically shared by both parents and are often reinforced by the complaints of the older non-ADHD siblings, grandparents, teachers, and school counselors. Often, by the time these parents consult with a therapist, their feelings of inadequacy have spread beyond parenting issues to other parts of their personal lives, and certainly into their marital relationship. Many parents, particularly full-time mothers, display clear symptoms of clinical depression, which reflect their sense of helplessness and of being "trapped with no escape." This depression may also be related to the disappointment discussed above, whereby many of these parents are grieving for the "lost" child they had imagined having. They will often express feeling cheated and angry, but sometimes have difficulty admitting these feelings because of a deeper vein of shame and guilt.

The Sibling Response

This is the stage where a growing sense of jealousy and rivalry between siblings and ADHD children erupts in open conflict. In the early evolution of these interactive dynamics, these feelings of jealousy and rivalry are more typically focused on the ADHD sibling whose behaviors are disruptive and interfere with normal family functioning, ultimately *reducing their time with, and attention from, their parents*. Many older non-ADHD siblings tell us that they do not look forward to doing anything as a family—be it going out to dinner, shopping, or going on vacations—because of the disruptiveness of their ADHD sibling. They also complain about the continual conflict that is present between their parents as they try to manage their ADHD sibling at home and in public places.

This rivalry for attention often spreads reciprocally throughout the entire sibling subsystem, such that family members sometimes come for therapy because one of the non-ADHD siblings has become "physical" and "abusive" toward the ADHD child, other siblings, or even a parent. This is a clear clinical example of how the initial behavioral symptoms of the ADHD child spread circularly throughout the family system and are then expressed or acted out by other members.

Often siblings feel that they are receiving less time with their parents. Their jealousy will emerge quickly as a rivalry with their ADHD brother or sister. If the parents do not respond to these early warning signs by balancing their time and attention with all of the children, greater sibling conflict will erupt within the entire nuclear system, conflict that is no longer just focused on the ADHD sibling. Many older siblings tell us that they were relieved when their ADHD sibling started school because then "Mom and Dad could come to my school" or "Mom had time to help me with my school work." Some of these older siblings even admit that they would sometimes fake being sick in order to stay home with their mother for the sheer pleasure of having her to themselves.

The Marital Response

The overall sense of frustration and anger can quickly spread into the marital relationship. It is the exceptional parents of ADHD children who are able to maintain patience and cooperative parenting during this early stage. As we have mentioned, clinicians need to recognize that the early frustrations of parenting an ADHD child are compounded developmentally by the fact that these parents are typically young adults in their mid- to later 20s who may have been married only 5 to 8 years. Clinical concerns cannot be focused solely on the ADHD child and associated parenting problems because these struggles threaten the core of this couple's communication resources and may have damaged their early bonding experiences. By this time in their marriage, the parents' need to focus time and energy on their ADHD child will have resulted in reduced personal and relationship privacy. These parents often tell us that "We rarely go out because we can't find anyone to stay with our son," or "The children fight so much when we're gone, we are afraid to leave them," or "Every time we sit down to talk, one or the other of the children has to sit in our laps or right between us. Even when we try to go into our bedroom or outside, they follow us there."

The dynamic that clinicians will observe here is clear: *the boundaries around the spousal subsystem are diffuse and poorly defined.* Gradually these parents lose the time alone and privacy they need for intimacy or even personal communication. The family becomes what is often referred to as a *child-focused family.* Much of their waking time together is spent discussing the children and trying to manage them. Even when they comply with the therapist's suggestion to go out to dinner without the children, much of their conversation revolves around the ADHD child or the children in general. Often their interactions become blatantly argumentative as the result of disputes over managing the children.

Many parents of young ADHD children, responding to a perceived sense of vulnerability in their child, become overprotective. Due to the countless problems that have marked these early years and the child's resulting low self-esteem, many parents are reluctant to allow sitters or extended family members to watch their ADHD child, even when the child is willing. The duality of resentment over the need for increased watchfulness coupled with this overprotectiveness often leads to considerable marital conflict, disruption, and disagreement.

STAGE 3: THE EARLY GRADE SCHOOL YEARS

As the ADHD child enters first grade and begins to engage in the basic educational tasks of learning reading, writing, and mathematics, the full range of ADHD difficulties begins to emerge. For the child who has struggled with her or his parents' and siblings' reactions to her or his impulsive and hyperactive behaviors, the onset of learning difficulties at this stage only reinforces an already low sense of self-esteem and lack of confidence. The clear overlay of emotional and psychological problems for the ADHD child begins to manifest in response to the frustrations of these early school years. In preschool the child was able to be more active, to play frequently, and to act somewhat impulsively without an excessively restrictive reaction from the teachers. However, in elementary school the tasks of sitting still at one's desk, paying attention, delaying gratification, and tolerating frustration are required. Children are expected to work silently at their desks and not to distract their fellow students. They are expected to pay attention, not interrupt, and follow directions without undue noise. These tasks and expectations are not easily met by most ADHD children. During these grade school years, the child may begin to see herself or himself as a failure. Observing other children meet the expectations of parents, teachers, and other adults, she or he will feel increasingly frustrated that she or he is unable to do so. It is in these years that ADHD children begin to feel different, inadequate, even stupid.

The Child's Experience

As children begin their grade school years, there is a gradual yet dramatic developmental shift in their primary social and interactional milieu from that of their family system to the new teacher- and peer-oriented systems of their school experiences. For the hyperactive child, this shift only adds another dimension of challenge and struggle: to try to contain his or her behaviors in these new settings with new teachers and new peers. For the predominantly inattentive child who has not struggled with serious early behavioral problems, these initial school experiences can become a source of new frustrations and even delays in learning basic skills such as reading, writing, and mathematics. Some ADHD children struggle with letters, numbers, and even handwriting as early as first grade. Nonhyperactive ADHD children may not manifest difficulties in these areas (particularly if they are intellectually bright) until the fifth to seventh grades.

Within the social context of these early school years, the ADHD child's impaired social skills and self-management difficulties become prominent. Many ADHD children at this age display significant immaturity, particularly in social skills. In grade school they may have trouble making friends. Some will frequently refuse to go to school, particularly if they have an overly protective parent. These children may be shy and quiet, which is often misinterpreted as unresponsiveness to their peers' and teachers' efforts to engage them. In contrast, the hyperactive children will simply frustrate and alienate peers who attempt to play with them, for they are often incapable of sharing toys or tolerating frustration, and they may impulsively hit a child who does not play the way they want to play. Over time, other children's mothers will prevent their child from playing with the impulsive or aggressive ADHD child because they are afraid that their own child will develop similar problem behaviors. Despite their often active and engaging traits, many of these young ADHD children experience lonely times and cannot understand why other children will not play with them, or why they are not allowed to go to their friends' houses to play. Unfortunately, because they are often shunned, many ADHD children at this stage have limited opportunities to learn more adaptive ways of playing with other children.

A third-grade boy, bright enough to qualify for most gifted programs, was brought to therapy by his parents, who described him as a "loner" who is often sad because he cannot make friends and feels that others do not like him. Nevertheless, he was imaginative, inventive, and self-reflective. He could quote passages from an encyclopedia he had been reading on scientific topics that caught his imagination. (This advanced reading was approved only after the therapist [SVE] negotiated it with his teacher, who had rigidly required that he read only second- and third-grade-level stories.) He drew pictures of rockets and cars not just in outline form, as most third-graders do, but complete with internal engines and gears. He was quite emotionally sensitive to his surroundings—for example, during thunderstorms he would hide under a table in his classroom.

In our play sessions he was highly likable. He was attentive and engaging with the therapist, always looking for verbal or mechanical challenges, and quick to suggest activities. When the therapist observed him at school, however, he was aggressive and competitive and challenged his playmates for attention. The energetic and engaging behaviors the therapist had experienced now took on a quality of pushiness and even rudeness. It was clear that many of his peers simply avoided him by either relocating their play or by ignoring his advances.

Depending on the severity of the child's symptoms, it will become apparent to the clinician (and many teachers) that general ego problems, including self-identity and self-esteem, are present by the third or fourth grades. Some children will simply be highly frustrated and discouraged. The predominantly inattentive ADHD children will begin to withdraw their investment in the educational process because they have difficulty performing expected tasks in the classroom and cannot understand why their friends can complete these tasks better and in less time. This early withdrawal is an attempt to defend themselves against what they perceive as an often relentless attack on their efforts to pay attention in the classroom, complete assignments, and pass tests. Their perception of being "under attack" is reinforced regularly by teachers, parents, siblings, grandparents, and even therapists. The role and responsibilities of the therapist are complicated by the multiple layers of stress. Educational struggles, parent–child and sibling conflicts, and growing self-esteem damage must be identified and ameliorated.

Many of these children in these early grade school years desperately want to behave better and try very hard to manage their impulses and adapt to the expectations of their parents and teachers—sadly, usually without success. Many children tell us, in essence, "I really try to pay attention [or listen better, or not clown around], but I just can't." Or they may say gravely, "Something must be wrong with me because I really want to stop getting in trouble, but it's like I'm someone else and can't make myself stop." It can be heartbreaking to hear how much many of these children want to please the adults around them and how unhappy they feel about their inability to do so. If the therapist plays too much of a corrective parenting role with the child, these underlying emotions may never be heard. Self-management is an impossible concept for many of these ADHD children, who do not have the slightest idea how to go about simple, everyday tasks that other children (and their teachers) take for granted.

The Parental Response

By the time the ADHD child is in the second or third grade, the parents of the hyperactive child have grown accustomed to calls from teachers and school counselors. Many feel that they need to defend themselves, or at least protect their child, from the increasing number of school complaints. They learn quickly that the preschool struggles they encountered with their hyperactive child did not magically disappear with the start of grade school and the managerial involvement of teachers.

The parents of ADHD children with predominantly inattention will begin to question whether their child is as bright as they had hoped or fantasized. It is very painful for parents to adjust their hopes for their child's future when they discover their first- and second-graders displaying difficulties remembering the alphabet and spelling simple words or reading basic stories. Many parents wonder secretly, "Maybe my child will not grow up to be successful, or even go to college." Suddenly their parenting role is blighted by a profound sense of discouragement and hopelessness.

The Protector and Critical Parent Roles

At this point, due to their ADHD child's academic and social struggles, many parents take on specifically identifiable roles that become clearly defined and lasting within the family system's structure. These roles can best be described as the *protector parent* and the *critical parent*. They evolve within a family system as a means of balancing the manner by which the family handles stress and crises. The critical parent displays excessive scrutiny, negative verbal feedback, and often relentless criticism regarding the child's problem behaviors and school difficulties. This critical parent can also become highly confrontational with the ADHD child, as well as functioning as an intimidating "enforcer." In some ADHD families, the task of verbally trying to control the child becomes exacerbated to the point where the parent is at risk of committing physical violence.

Parents who assume the protector role feel sorry for their child's struggles; can identify, at least at times, with the child's frustration and pain; and often mediate, defend, or block negative feedback directed at the child. The protector parent intervenes consistently in a rescuing manner when the other parent or siblings "pick on" the ADHD child, even if punishment is deserved. This parent will also intervene in the school setting by trying to "explain away" her or his child's misbehaviors and/or failures. Frequently blame is shifted to the teacher. This protector parent is one who may arrive weekly at the principal's office complaining that the teacher does not "understand" the child and/or is "not being fair."

The role of protector parent is not gender-specific. Sometimes it is the parent who also has ADHD and now identifies and sympathizes with the behaviors of this child. Such a parent tells teachers and therapists, "But I did the same thing when I was his age," as if this explanation offers a solution in itself. The protector role can also be played by the non-ADHD parent, whether mother or father, who feels sorry for her or his child's apparent victimization by the ADHD parent's impatient and reactive behaviors, or by the school's persistent complaints. Sometimes it is the full-time mother who becomes the protector because she is around the child's struggles all day; other times, it is the full-time mother who becomes the critical parent simply because she spends most of her time managing and mediating conflicts at home.

A mother of four children had become the protector of her eldest son, John, by the time he had entered the first grade. He was 11-years-old and in the sixth grade when the family was referred to us (CAE). He had never been diagnosed with ADHD. His academic success during his early grade school years had diminished dramatically since the beginning of fifth grade. The mother remembered a teacher "in the first or second grade" who had told her that John was having difficulty with math and might have "some attention problems." But she took no action in response to these observations at that point. John was still having difficulty with math, and now also falling behind in spelling and reading. Halfway through the first semester of the sixth grade he began expressing many somatic complaints and was chronically absent from school—a pattern that had been present for several years but had become prominent the prior spring. The mother told the therapist that she had indulged these behaviors and absences through the spring semester of the fifth grade because "he was having such a difficult time." Now the pediatrician had referred John for a clinical evaluation because there was no medical basis for his physical complaints and resulting absences from school.

When the mother arrived for her initial appointment, she said her husband had been too busy to come. Later it was learned that she had not even told her husband about the appointment because she did not want the therapist (CAE) "to hear the bad side" about John. She said that her husband (the apparent "critical" parent) was angrier and more impatient with both the child's and her own behaviors. She explained that she had three other children, 9, 6, and 4 years old. The 4-year-old stayed at home with her, and John, she admitted, enjoyed staying at home "to help her out during the day."

The mother reported that over the prior 6 weeks, much to her husband's displeasure, she had let the child stay home on average 2 to 3 days each week. Later it was also discovered that the father only knew about a few of these absences. On the days that the child did attend school, the mother would send the other two children off on the bus at the normal time and then take John to school in the car. She and her son would sit in the car until the bell rang; he had few friends and had felt "uncomfortable" being by himself on the playground area since several children had "picked on" him. He had also refused to eat lunch in the school cafeteria, so for the past several weeks the mother would take herself and her 4-year-old with her to the school and eat lunch with Johnny in the waiting area of the principal's office.

School refusal at this age is fairly uncommon. Clinically, a typical response to this pattern would be to look for signs of depression and phobic reactions in the child. The clinician would also notice John's clearly excessive dependency on his mother and the relative safety that he felt at home, as well as the mother's reciprocal protectiveness and reliance on him. The clinician would look for problems and/or events that may have been threatening for the child at school. Therapeutic interventions for a child of this age might focus on individual therapy, perhaps supportive and/or cognitive group therapy with other students, and some background interviews with the parents. However, if the therapist simply treated the school refusal behaviors for this child, he or she would never address the underlying etiological issues for both John and his family.

Exploring the presenting clinical issues from a broader systemic perspective, the therapist would review the child's and the family's social and educational histories. Of course, right away, the therapist would not be comfortable with excuses about a father's absence in the initial interview. The mother's passing comment in the initial interview—"a teacher in the first or second grade said he may have some attention problems"—would be a red flag. In the case of John, further evaluation, based on the parents' reports, a review of school records, and testing data would reveal that John displayed early and continuing attention and distractibility problems, with serious visual processing deficits that clearly inhibited his skills with math and reading.

At the end of this initial session the therapist insisted that the father come in with the mother for the next interview, whereupon the mother tearfully acknowledged that she had never told her husband about the appointment. (Related clinical issues regarding the participation of both parents in the initial interviews will be discussed in Chapter 6.)

However, the mother's perception about her husband was correct. It was clear that he had assumed a critical and even confrontational role toward John, blaming the child for being "lazy" and "not listening." He justified his criticalness as his "taking on the disciplinarian role of the family since my wife does not do it." He also belittled his wife for treating John "like a baby" and for "not letting him grow up." It was difficult for the therapist to remain neutral here and not be pulled into the family's interactional dynamics. This can happen quite suddenly for the less experienced therapist, who may respond automatically to the emotional drama of the interactional system—in this case, attacker versus protector and victimized child. The therapist felt himself being pulled to defend not only John but also the mother from her husband's attacks.

However, by staying focused on the broader systemic picture, the therapist could acknowledge that the father's critical attacks were not without foundation. Mother, as the protector, had entered into a secret alliance with John to the exclusion of both her husband and the other children. The multilevel systemic issues are quite clear in this case. The father's reactions were not just to the child's struggles in school but to the clearly divergent parenting approaches and the breach of trust and honesty that he felt in both the parenting and marital relationship with his wife.

A subsequent sibling session revealed clearly that the other children resented the time their mother spent with John and his special status with her. They were also angry with their father, who had withdrawn from many parenting roles due to his frustration and disputes with his wife. The specific presenting symptoms—John's many somatic complaints and school absences—were merely the "tip of the iceberg." Staying home during the day gave John a sense of safety: he could not fail or be criticized at school if he was not there. Of course, he was also safe from his father's attacks since he was at work. He had the covert assurance from his mother that his home would remain a safe and protective place.

Unfortunately, this mother did not seek therapy for her child until she finally felt overwhelmed, and she acknowledged that she was beginning to feel guilty because she was ignoring and neglecting the other three children and she did not know how to deal with her husband's growing anger. In the tearful second interview, for which the father was present, the mother acknowledged: "Johnny is so much like I was when I was his age in school. I had all of the same problems. I hated school, but my parents made me go. I didn't want to do that to him."

This case is an effective example of the broad level of interactional dynamics that can emerge in a family around symptoms of ADHD. Of course, the systemic patterns surround, and often camouflage, the ADHD symptoms before they are recognized. Specifically, it demonstrates the powerful influence of the ADHD disorder on the identity and functioning of every family member, as well as the complex interactive and potentially dysfunctional roles that can evolve between spouses.

Paradoxically, the critical parent is often the parent with undiagnosed ADHD. More often, however, the critical parent is simply the one who demands more structure and discipline within the family. In the former case, the parent's impatience and reactivity to her or his own difficulties may be directed at the child's disappointing performances and failures in school. The critical parent may become unyielding in her or his demands on the child to "study more," "do better," and "pay attention." This establishes the reciprocal pattern in the parenting subsystem whereby the other parent, whether or not he or she has ADHD traits, will take on the role of the protector by intervening and mediating so that the child does not feel even more overwhelmed. We consistently observe in many ADHD families that the greater the degree of critical and/or attacking behavior by one parent, the greater will be the degree of protective response by the other parent.

These contrasting dynamics, as they are observed by the therapist, can become a fatal trap for many clinicians who become seduced by the emotional drama of the system. If the therapist intervenes in an attempt to protect the child, rather than objectively assessing and intervening with the broader system's dynamics, the risk of alienating the critical parent is great. This can result in the therapist's loss of credibility and power for continuing work with the family.

We have also observed that the greater the degree of protection experienced by the ADHD child from a parent, the greater will be that child's continuing sense of dependency on both the protective parent and the family milieu in general. This establishes the intergenerational transmission of dependency that we identified in genograms in Chapter 4.

Scapegoating Pattern

An alternate family dynamic that is present in many ADHD families is the *scapegoating* of the ADHD child. When this occurs both parents align themselves against the ADHD child, creating a negative and critical focus toward the child's problematic behaviors as well as the child's role in the family. In this process of scapegoating the troubled child, other members of the family, including siblings and grandparents, all develop a shared perception of the child that is highly negative. They typically characterize this child as bad, or mean, or "the problem." There is often a shared family belief that if this scapegoated child would "just behave" or "grow up," then all would be fine in the family.

Scapegoating occurs in many families for many reasons and is *always* hurtful. When directed at an ADHD child, scapegoating can be devastating. The child feels totally overwhelmed and essentially abandoned; no one in the family really cares about her or him. There is no protector or mediator in the family to intervene or soften the attacks. This scapegoating dynamic produces the rageful, potentially violent, reaction seen in young adolescents who have conduct disorder. Often this pattern of scapegoating contaminates the child's school experiences, for it is replicated and thereby reinforced by teachers and principals. As the ADHD children of this stage get older, the scapegoating pattern can also follow them into their social and peer interactions, as "friends" and even the parents of their peers point the finger of blame and accusation.

Combination Pattern

Some ADHD families may display a combination of these two patterns: what begins in a family as scapegoating provokes the emergence of a protector to rescue the ADHD child. This protector role may appear during certain developmental or age-specific periods, such as kindergarten and first grade. It may also appear only in certain contexts, such as when the child is ill or playing sports. In families characterized by intense scapegoating, this protection may be highly circumscribed—for example, the child is protected from attacks by siblings but not from attacks by the other parent (or significantly less so). Often in these scapegoating systems the quasi-protective parent will, under pressure, align with the critical parent against the ADHD child.

Most parents experience ambivalent feelings toward their difficult child. On the one hand, parents feel a special need to nurture this child whom they know has an especially difficult time in school and with friends. On the other hand, they are often so frustrated and discouraged by the constant struggles with the child that they have little patience left for being nurturant and loving. It is somewhat easier for parents to exercise patience with the inattentive ADHD child, who often appears more anxious and dependent. With the hyperactive–impulsive child, the parents' patience and tolerance levels are sorely tested and they will often vacillate between being overly punitive and being overly protective. This inconsistency only exacerbates the child's symptoms and leads to a confusing and distressing uncertainty about how the parent really feels and how they will respond.

The Sibling Response

Siblings often respond to their ADHD counterpart with anger and isolation. As they grow increasingly intolerant of their sibling's disruptive behaviors and the inordinate amount of attention the ADHD child receives from the parents, siblings of all ages find ways to express their discontentment. Younger siblings may display jealousy, whining, and clinging behaviors as indicators of feeling neglected. Older siblings tend to be more angry and argumentative, and they often confront their ADHD sibling as well as their parents. As they reach adolescence, these siblings begin to see their younger ADHD sibling as the enemy. They often express to us outright hatred and even wishes that their sibling would die.

The non-ADHD siblings experience a sense of rejection by their parents, believing that they are simply not as important as their troubled sister or brother. They begin to isolate themselves from the ADHD child and they may also become withdrawn and distant from each other. Parents who overprotect the ADHD child tend to see their non-ADHD children as being more capable of shouldering responsibility and meeting expectations. Thus, in disputes involving the ADHD child and a sibling, often the parent will expect far more from the non-ADHD child, even a younger one. The parents may also punish the non-ADHD child more quickly or harshly, stating, "You can help it but he can't" or "You know better but she doesn't." The unfairness of the parent's response further alienates and isolates these siblings from the ADHD child and reinforces the scapegoating process by siblings.

The Marital Response

The dramatic protector–critical parent dynamic that we have discussed clearly invades and defines many marital relationships. Even though it is played out toward the ADHD child, the oppositional roles polarize the marital interaction and set the stage for chronic unresolvable and adversarial confrontations between the spouses. The sense of maintaining a team approach to parenting that united spouses in the earlier years will have dissipated by this stage, leaving husband and wife openly at odds with each other. They may disagree on discipline, structure, homework, the role of the school, and the child's abilities both educationally and socially.

Even spouses who have not fallen into the protector–critical parent role dichotomy will begin to experience high levels of stress by this stage, which invariably undermines their communication and their intimacy with one another. Parents who constantly argue over their child will find little satisfaction in either emotional or sexual intimacy. Gradually they begin to withdraw emotional support for one another. This leads to increasingly poor or nonexistent communication and further emotional distancing, wherein spouses share less mutual time and fewer activities together. The father may stay at work later and later, while the mother feels increasingly trapped by longer periods of time alone at home to struggle with the difficult child *and* the growing resentment and anger among the siblings. The father's isolation from the family may be a result of his feeling pushed out of the parenting role or it may simply reflect his desire to avoid chronic fighting with his wife. He may extend the range of his withdrawal to include avoiding family activities, outings, and even vacations. Over a period of time this isolation will begin to undermine the couple's communication and intimacy. In some cases this distancing in the marital relationship leads to another scapegoating pattern wherein the wife aligns with the unhappy children, making her husband into the "bad guy." This creates a coalition that further distances the father/husband and exacerbates the level of marital discord.

STAGE 4: THE LATER GRADE SCHOOL YEARS

As the ADHD child reaches fourth, fifth, and sixth grades, the range of presenting symptoms becomes more complex for the clinician. The disruptive ADHD behaviors and increasing levels of personal and academic failures and frustrations of the hyperactive–impulsive children begin to form *conduct disorder patterns* at home and at school. Their reactivity becomes more confrontational and directed first toward objects, then siblings, then peers, then teachers, then parents. As they become older and physically larger, the types of disruptions that characterized their early years now make a more serious impact and get them into deeper trouble more readily. Teachers report more threatening and/or defiant behaviors, as well as more fights at school. Even the more inattentive-type ADHD child will often begin to display more reactive and oppositional behaviors in this stage. They often have an intense dislike for school by this time and believe that they will never be capable of succeeding. They may attempt to get out of going to school any way possible. These are also the years when other types of emotional difficulties appear concurrently with ADHD, such as anxiety, obsessive–compulsive, depressive, and conduct disorders.

The Child's Experience

While some ADHD children exhibit a subtler range of generalized symptoms, many display clearly diagnosable comorbid disorders. The inattentive ADHD child often displays more emotional symptoms at this age, particularly those of anxiety and depression. These children recognize that school is becoming increasingly difficult. Though they are often told that they are bright, they are not able to perform as successfully as their friends or their siblings. These experiences serve to exacerbate their personal frustrations and to entrench their growing sense of failure. Many children at this stage are referred for therapy not because of school failure or ADHD symptoms, but because of anxiety or depression. The anxiety can take many forms: unusual fears, panic disorders, simple phobias (school phobia is especially common), and obsessive–compulsive disorder (OCD).

A 12-year-old girl was referred to us because the mother was concerned that her daughter was developing an eating disorder. The child would eat only certain, very specific items and would not let any food on her plate touch any other food. She was quite thin but still believed she needed to lose weight. In school she was a perfectionist who had to have absolutely perfect schoolwork.

She would recopy a paper 10 times, if necessary, to make it look perfect. This often meant that she spent 5 or 6 hours at night doing her homework and would not go to bed until very late. She would be very upset if she did not get A's on her assignments and would obsess about why she had not done better.

In talking with the mother, it became apparent to us that this child had great difficulty following what the teacher was explaining and also felt frustrated when she missed something the teacher had said. She put great effort into paying attention, so much so that she was exhausted by the end of each school day. The therapist (SVE) recommended that she be evaluated but the school refused to do any testing, since they perceived her as "an excellent student." She was tested privately. The results of the tests supported the clinical observations that she had the inattentive form of ADHD and was working at full capacity trying to overcome the difficulties this presented for her.

Although she was very bright, she tried to compensate for her ADHD symptoms by her efforts to be "perfect"—which resulted in constant anxiety about everything in her life and physical and emotional exhaustion. After this was explained to the school, and accommodations were made for her, many of her OCD symptoms vanished, as did the signs of an eating disorder. With the help of medication and family therapy she was finally able "to give herself a break" and reduce the pressure she was applying to herself daily. It was fortunate that this family sought help before the additional symptoms evolved into a full-scale eating disorder. The family also had an older daughter who had been diagnosed with ADHD some years earlier, but neither the teacher, nor a prior therapist, nor the parents themselves recognized an association between these sisters' symptoms.

These children often have other emotional difficulties that mask the ADHD symptoms and often fool both physicians and school personnel. In a general clinical assessment of children this age, it is important to be aware that, when school struggles are a part of the overall pattern of difficulties, an underlying ADHD pattern may be present.

The Parental Response

Many parents feel a sense of helplessness and inadequacy in dealing with their ADHD child and attempting to manage related issues with their other children. Some of these parents talk about feeling so out of control or overwhelmed that they begin to second-guess themselves as parents. Some begin to yell at their children as a way of trying to regain control, or simply to vent their frustrations. These parents focus on their angry and punitive feelings toward both their ADHD child and their other children. They may react more sharply to one of their non-ADHD children, losing patience quickly. Everyday issues take on far greater significance when there is a pervasive sense of "losing control of the family." These parenting and control issues can cause frustrations to spiral out of control in a manner that clearly affects—and sometimes endangers—all of the children.

Scapegoating reaches even greater proportions at this stage. The potential for violence increases as the ADHD child and siblings grow older and more unmanageable, further compounding the chronic frustrations that continue, without relief, for the parents. In some families, punitiveness and frustration turns into physical abuse, at first directed toward the ADHD child and later toward the other children. Certainly, in most families, the verbal abuse and criticism directed toward the ADHD child rises sharply during this time.

This stage is a critical period for both assessment and clinical interventions. Children who have not been diagnosed with ADHD by the end of this stage will carry their symptoms and behaviors, as well as the negative responses from their families, into the more complicated life of middle school, puberty, and early adolescence. Similarly, ADHD children who have not received effective and coordinated therapeutic and educational interventions will continue to struggle with even greater expectations as they enter middle school. If programs are developed for early therapeutic and educational identification of ADHD, they must be in place and effective before the close of this stage.

The Sibling Response

Siblings may feel increasing alienation from their ADHD sister/ brother and, eventually, from their family in general. Older siblings are now adolescents; they may contemplate moving out of the home to get away from their ADHD sibling and the chronic level of conflict in the household. We have heard these adolescents plead with their parents to let them live with a friend or even to leave town to live with a relative. Many parents often cannot understand the piercing level of frustration felt by their non-ADHD children.

When the scapegoating pattern is part of the family dynamics, the verbal confrontations and pushing and shoving by siblings that characterized the early years can now quickly escalate to physical threats and hitting. The danger here is that the reactive and impulsive tendencies of the ADHD child will "fan the flames" of these confrontations to a level where even the parents will have difficulty intervening to protect the children.

Long-term conflict will have lasting effects on non-ADHD adolescent siblings. Gradually these feelings are transferred from the ADHD sibling exclusively to their parents. Most of the adolescent siblings tell us of their disillusionment with and even rage toward their parents. Many feel that they were blamed unfairly for everyday confrontations, while their ADHD sibling escaped punishment. Many feel that they "put up with," "tolerated," and "lived with the embarrassment" of their ADHD sibling, but suffered without gaining the respect and gratitude from their parents that they deserved. Gradually these adolescents may *withdraw their affect and identification from the ADHD sibling, from their other siblings, and eventually from their parents and family in general.* They simply differentiate early from the family and try to lead more independent lives by affiliating with high school friends and activities. Many of these siblings leave home with a sense of sadness and grief, feeling that they have lost an important part of their growing-up and family experience.

The Marital Response

The patterns that we have described in the marital dynamics of the earlier stages continue to grow and escalate in this stage. What we often observe here is that the *high levels of conflict become generalized from parental issues into broader everyday life interactions.* These generalized conflicts may appear in parenting the other children, in financial discussions, in leisure time activities, and in sexual intimacy. Often the entire marital relationship is in chaos. For many marriages this long-term pattern of stress, conflict, and frustration leads to substantial distancing between the two partners. Many parents tell us "We have not taken a vacation together in years," or "We rarely go out to dinner any more," or "We haven't made love in months [sometimes years]." This lack of personal connection may result in more time spent at work or in activities away from one another, as well as a greater frequency of extramarital relationships. The children are quite aware of their parents' conflicts and often talk about the unhappiness and turmoil that they experience in their parents.

STAGE 5: THE MIDDLE AND HIGH SCHOOL YEARS

For most children, the shift from the relative stability and expectable safety of grade school to the increased demands and responsibilities of middle school can be unnerving. For ADHD children this transition is even more problematic. They are now faced with six to eight different teachers, multiple classrooms, increased social demands, teachers who will never know them as well as their fifth- or sixth-grade teachers, and teachers who expect more and give more homework. For many undiagnosed inattentive-type ADHD children who are bright, the underlying symptoms of the disorder will finally become more apparent. Many parents of such children tell us that our diagnosis simply cannot be right because their child "never struggled in grade school, the teachers always liked him [her], and he [her] was never in trouble." They often conclude: "It must be the teenage thing," or "It must be because he [she] is hanging out with new friends who never study or do their homework either," or "The teachers just don't explain things to him [her]."

The clinician, parents, and teachers should recognize that this transition for ADHD children to middle school presents dramatically new logistics and expectations that can be critical to the child's future educational success and ongoing self-esteem. Helping them develop a sense of structure and organization to manage the chaos of their new experiences and demands is crucial. Many older undiagnosed ADHD adolescents that we do not see until they are juniors or seniors in high school can date the onset of their struggles in school from these beginning difficulties in middle school. For example, one high school senior, who had just been diagnosed with ADHD and who was struggling to get grades of D's and C's, said angrily, "Why didn't anyone figure this out then [in seventh grade]? At least I would have been able to have a future."

The Adolescent's Experience

The struggles of the ADHD child in grade school, both behaviorally and educationally, may seem mild compared to the form they often take in adolescence. Patterns of reactivity can evolve into intimidation and violence; discouragement may deepen into clinical depression; lack of confidence can develop into fear; early struggles with letters and numbers can escalate into school failure, regular truancy, and eventual dropping out. The clinician must recognize that at this stage the ADHD adolescent can potentially display a *broad range of generalized dysfunctional behaviors that exist beyond the typical cluster of ADHD symptoms.*

These additional problematic behaviors develop because of the interplay of the adolescent's experiences with puberty and physical development, the expectations for social skills and educational success, and their gradual separation from the safety of their family milieu. The associated ADHD symptoms and the continuing academic and behavioral struggles exacerbate the adolescent's frustration and further lower his or her self-esteem. The interaction of all these factors tends to render the ADHD adolescent at risk for other dysfunctional symptoms, ranging from anxiety to depression to oppositional to conduct-disordered behaviors.

For many ADHD adolescents, academic struggles become more dramatic in the first year of middle school and evolve into chronic school failure. These experiences of failure may prompt habitual truancy and then dropping out of school all together. The research cited in Chapter 2 reported high levels of comorbid oppositional defiant and conduct disorders behaviors in ADHD adolescents. Many of these adolescents are not only frustrated and unhappy, they have begun to feel that they "just don't fit" either in school or in their families. Their low self-esteem is continually reinforced in most areas of their lives, and they feel that they only receive criticism and expressions of dissatisfaction from their parents. A number of these discouraged ADHD adolescents will turn to substance abuse. Some do so for excitement and adventure, others for self-medication. Many high school ADHD students who have been successfully medicated with stimulants can describe how they began using amphetamines or even cocaine in their middle school years because it made them feel more relaxed or settled. Some of these students even point out that these drugs were more effective and satisfying for them than alcohol. Certainly, this involvement with drugs can lead many adolescents into more delinquent behaviors and community conflicts, not to mention increased levels of confrontation and reactivity at home with their parents and siblings. Some of these adolescents may give up and run away.

It is difficult to predict specific patterns of comorbid symptoms that may occur among ADHD adolescents because there are so many possible symptom combinations. The ones who have displayed more hyperactive and impulsive behaviors may be more prone to conduct disorder in adolescence. However, we also see many primarily inattentive ADHD adolescents who, due to their history of school failures and other frustrations, show oppositional defiant behaviors both toward their family and at school. Some ADHD adolescents may be more prone to depression. These patterns appear in part to be a function of the prior family dynamics. If there is a history of depression in the family, an ADHD adolescent might also display depression. If there has been a history of anger, punitiveness, and threats of violence in the family, an ADHD adolescent is likely to display conduct disorder.

One of the few exceptions to this pattern occurs when ADHD adolescents, both males and females, have athletic skills or prior success in sports-related activities. These adolescents can still find a measure of motivation, optimism, and success in this theater of their lives. This is particularly true of the hyperactive–impulsive ADHD adolescents. If they can channel their energy and intensity into a sports activity, they may be able to find an area of success for themselves. Many ADHD adults will tell us, reflectively, that the only positive thing they remember about high school was that they "made the basketball team" or that they "got a letter in volleyball" or they were "good at soccer." We have worked with many hyperactive ADHD adolescents who, in their early years, enjoyed sports but had difficulty "getting along with other members of the team or the coaches." Unfortunately, some ADHD adolescents give up on sports experiences. Sometimes we try to refocus their interests in the direction of other sports that are based more on individual skills and not dependent upon team interaction.

A high school freshman, recently diagnosed with ADHD, hyperactive–impulsive type, was floundering in school. He had been kicked off his soccer team the previous year, which had caused him to give up all sports activities. One of the authors (CAE), who saw him in therapy, explored other options with him that might help him remain active rather than indulge his angry desire to relinquish participation in all sports. He was somewhat short for his age but he was well developed physically. He could have played linebacker on a football team, but he certainly would have had difficulty in terms of team members interaction and cooperation, just as he did on his soccer team. After some discussion over several weeks, wrestling was considered as a possible option, since his father had wrestled in high school.

His mother was cautious because she saw wrestling as a "violent sport like football." His father, who had been successful in both soccer and wrestling in his youth, eventually convinced his wife that it would be "worth a try." The boy was accepted on the freshman team that year. He adapted well to the training and the combative nature of the sport. The coach tolerated some of his disruptive behavior because he valued the boy's intensity and leadership abilities. In practice he could win matches against team members who outweighed him by as much as 30 to 40 pounds. The high levels of energy and intensity that he brought to the wrestling ring came as a surprise to everyone, his therapist included.

By agreement with his parents and due to the school's policies, he knew that he had to keep his grades up to continue wrestling. By his senior year he was getting mostly C's and an occasional B on his report card. By the end of the wrestling season in his senior year he was ranked second in the state for his weight class. He had even been approached by two small state college coaches who had no scholarships to offer but who invited him to enroll and "walk on" for their wrestling teams. He felt good about himself, and the success that he had achieved as a wrestler helped him finish high school without any further display of conduct problems. At the time of his graduation he conveyed considerably more maturity. He was able to express his appreciation to his parents for their support of his wrestling, adding that they "finally learned that I could be successful at something."

Unfortunately, many ADHD adolescents, especially those without hyperactive traits, may not have the level of intensity or competitiveness necessary to be successful, as the boy described above was. Nevertheless, the clinician and the school counselor need to pursue other possible alternatives. Support from his or her parents is also critical to any ADHD adolescent who is grappling with the possibility of trying new endeavors and taking risks in untried areas. If they assume that their parents will continue to be critical of them and expect failure, then they will not pursue these new experiences. The goal is to find a successful nonacademic experience for ADHD students that will serve to offset and balance their struggles in the classroom. Therapists and parents should nurture and special skill, talent, or interest that an ADHD adolescent may possess, with the object of helping that adolescent experience some sense of success. Sports is only one area to explore. For those not interested in sports, artistic pursuits, music, or theater activities may provide the ADHD adolescent with a venue in which they can feel successful, even special and unique. It has been our experience that ADHD adolescents are more successful in creative and active pursuits that provide stimulation and sustain their interest.

The ADHD trait of *hyperfocusing* is associated primarily with adult diagnoses, and it may not be recognized in adolescents. This trait, the capacity of many individuals with ADHD to focus narrowly and exclusively on a singular activity that is uniquely stimulating and challenging for them, is confusing to many parents as well as to the ADHD individuals themselves. For example, parents told us that they could not imagine how their son could have ADHD since "he sits for 3 hours without moving in front of the computer." An ADHD adult electrical engineer said that he never considered the possibility that he had an attention problem because he spent all day designing complex computer programs. An ADHD physician reported that he felt "at home and stimulated" with the crises in the hospital's emergency room. Paradoxically, this same physician struggled to sustain his interest and attention when playing games with his young children. Like the physician, many ADHD adults recall their difficulties with inattention and distractibility in most settings, never recognizing that their hyperfocusing resource actually aided them in accomplishing a certain task in a more thorough and efficient fashion than their colleagues.

In general, this resource allows many ADHD individuals to restrict and/or ignore all external influences and distractions for considerable periods of time. It is demonstrated in the child who can sit still and play computer games for hours, often not "hearing" the telephone ring or his mother's requests, but who cannot stay focused in the classroom; in the fighter pilot who can outmaneuver most other pilots in the air, but cannot complete reports and paperwork on the ground; in the emergency room physician who can make quick and accurate diagnostic judgments and lifesaving interventions with trauma cases but cannot sit quietly on the floor to play with his young children; the athlete who excels with high energy and competitiveness throughout a game but who cannot relax at home and has little patience with her children.

Obviously this hyperfocusing trait has both positive and negative features, but its negative side has received most of the attention. In working with ADHD adolescents, it can be extremely helpful to label it as a strength, even a "secret asset." Many adolescents respond well to the therapist's identification of this trait as a resource that "no one else has." We have successfully steered many ADHD adolescents toward activities such as computer clubs, chess clubs, marching bands, and the like. These are all areas where a potential for hyperfocusing can be experienced in a beneficial way. For example, one eighth-grade student we treated, who was getting grades of D in mathematics, became so proficient with computer operations and programming after reluctantly joining an afterschool computer club that his instructor helped him get a summer job assisting a public library in computerizing its entire catalog operations.

This hyperfocusing resource can be used to therapeutically "reframe" an adolescent's difficult ADHD symptoms in a more positive light. We often tell these adolescents stories about ADHD adults who have become quite successful in a variety of careers because they are able to utilize their hyperfocusing resources. Our reframing strategy takes the form of exploring, defining, and emphasizing the positive aspects of the adolescent's behaviors. With experience, the therapist can learn to recognize and identify both personality-related and cognitive resources of the ADHD adolescent, framing them as positive attributes that she or he can build upon.

Many ADHD adolescents struggle with the problematic combination of typical adolescent mood swings exacerbated by their impulsivity and volatility. Their impulsivity may lead them toward more reckless experimentation in a variety of areas, including sexuality, truancy, substance abuse, and gang-related activities. Certainly, a central therapeutic goal is helping the adolescent to become more self-aware, to learn accommodation skills to be more successful in the classroom, and to find social activities that are satisfying—all of which should help improve self-esteem, nurture a better overall attitude, and promote better judgments. Unfortunately, difficulties in making sound social judgments will follow many ADHD adolescents into their adult lives.

The Parental Response

By the time an ADHD child has reached adolescence, parental struggles have often heated to the boiling point. The lesser offenses of the young ADHD child become more serious now in the broader community, educationally and legally. For many parents of ADHD adolescents, this stage signals real concerns for the social and educational futures of their children. Parents who once dreamed of their child becoming a doctor or lawyer now share with us their worries about whether he or she will even finish high school. They also worry about "losing further control" of their child via drugs and delinquency, and about the concomitant potential for legal consequences.

At this point in their lives many parents are subjected to greater external pressures from the school, the community, and even legal sources regarding their ADHD adolescents. Many parents are burdened by an overwhelming sense of embarrassment about their child's failures and/or conduct. Most also suffer feeling inadequate as parents in the eyes of their own parents.

As ADHD adolescents' behaviors become more dramatic, the scapegoating phenomena continues to escalate. Often the scapegoating becomes more blatantly focused on the delinquency and failures of the ADHD adolescent, which are routinely proclaimed by older and younger siblings as well as intergenerational family members. The risk for physical abuse and/or conflict turning into violence is high at this stage on all fronts: from parents (particularly the critical parent), siblings, and the ADHD adolescent, not to mention his or her classmates.

For some parents, these concerns will continue throughout their child's high school experiences and even after the adolescent has left home. However, for other parents, we have observed a different pattern that emerges toward the end of their adolescent's high school experience. These parents, who are particularly hurt by their sense of parental failure, begin to withdraw from their ADHD adolescent. Many finally realize that they have neglected their other children and begin to shift their parental focus onto them, sometimes for the first time. Some simply "throw up their hands," declaring to anyone who will listen that they have done all that they could do. Many parents confide in us privately that if their ADHD child gets into legal trouble, they will "just let it happen, even if it means ending up in jail." The angrier parents might even hope that someone the courts will take over responsibility for their child. Some go so far as to state, "If he [she] gets arrested, we will not hire an attorney."

The Sibling Response

The potential for confrontations, even physical violence, toward the ADHD sibling continues to increase in many families throughout this stage. Many of the siblings, particularly the younger ones who are approaching puberty and adolescence, begin to act out on their own.

Their frustrations with their ADHD sibling and the conflict they experience at home may cause them to express their unhappiness toward their peers or teachers at school. Some will become confrontational with parents. Others will get into fights at school. Many of these siblings will tell us in essence: "No one listens to me at home and no one makes my brother behave. I feel so much tension that when someone at school says something to me, I just go off on them" or, "My sister gets away with everything—nobody can control her, she always gets what she wants, so I figured I might as well be the same way."

At this stage the older siblings are finishing their final years in high school. They are more independent and perhaps have differentiated themselves from their families as protection from the turmoil at home. Many are successful academically and/or athletically and tend to look down on their struggling ADHD sibling. They have their own friends and are looking ahead to escaping from the family and being on their own, whether it be working or going to college. By this stage they have withdrawn, both physically and emotionally, from their siblings and parents. In fact, many of these older siblings are reluctant to attend family therapy sessions because they feel so disconnected from the issues and problems at home. Others will tell us that they just do not want to be reminded of what goes on at home. Sometimes their parents are troubled because they no longer talk to them about their social lives or plans after graduation.

The Marital Response

Parents of ADHD adolescents are now 15 to 20 years into their marriages. The *empty nest syndrome,* parental grief because their children have grown up and left home, is not typically present in these families. In fact, the sadness experienced by these parents in their personal lives is much more likely to reflect their sense of parental failure. For some, there is a clear sense of relief that their parenting days are, at last, ending. The marital relationships of these spouses ranges from extremely distant and emotionally cut off to open rage and betrayal. Whether distant or rageful, both responses are spawned by disappointment, anger, and deep discouragement that culminates in a sense of marital failure. Many of these spouses face separation and/or divorce. For some divorce has already occurred. Many spouses express to us their sense of personal alienation, not just from their partners but from their extended family life. Many grieve over the irrevocable loss of happy and productive times with their other children and the love and companionship of their partner. By this stage many of these spouses display their own psychopathology, which may range from anxiety and mood disorders to substance abuse.

We have worked with many ADHD parents in marital therapy and have found that constructive changes *can* be made; it is not necessarily too late. It is a difficult clinical process because, even as parenting responsibilities are waning, the long-term accumulation of frustration and alienation needs to be cleared out of the way. For most of these spouses, their struggles with a different and unmanageable child began in the first 2 or 3 years of their marriages. Nevertheless, many of the couples do have the personal resources to reclaim their original attraction and caring for one another. But others have simply told us, "Too much has happened, and I don't think I love him anymore," or "Even if she changed, I'm not sure it would make any difference," or "I'm just too tired to imagine building a new relationship."

Many parents who look forward to their ADHD child leaving home also feel guilty, so much so that they may push their child to consider staying at home to go to college (and thereby assuage their consciences). However, other parents are adamant about their child becoming independent and finding a way of living away from home. Some of these parents have harbored a fantasy for years that after the ADHD adolescent leaves home, their marriage will automatically improve and they will be able to do the things together as a couple that they have never been able to do. But other parents fantasize about leaving the family and their partner, too, perhaps envisioning new partners after a divorce.

These feelings are not always present for the parent who has played a protective role in relation to the ADHD child. The more anxious, inattentive ADHD adolescent may not be ready to leave home after graduating from high school. As we discussed earlier, the greater the degree of parental protectiveness, the greater will be the ADHD adolescent's dependency on the family. In this developmental stage the dependency translates into poor differentiation and limited self-confidence. By now, some may have tried—and failed—to move out of the family home. The parents of these children are often very anxious and worried about their adolescent's ability to live away from them and are therefore reluctant to allow the child to participate in dorm living or to move into an apartment.

The natural clinical inclination would be to support and encourage the adolescent's normal drive for separation and to help the parents to adjust to this change and positively anticipate their emancipation. If this position is presented prematurely, however, the therapist may quickly lose the respect and confidence of the parents. Care and patience is needed when working with these dynamics in marital therapy when ADHD issues have been present historically for these spouses. It is important to understand that the potential family crisis now is not just about an adolescent leaving home: it is really about the parents finally facing their own internal struggles throughout 18 or more years of parenting an ADHD child. Not only do they need to support the adolescent in separating, but they also need to look at their own lives after years of ADHD parenting. Many spouses feel a continuing need to overprotect and monitor their ADHD child, and at the same time harbor an apprehension that there may not be anything left in their marriage if they are home alone with their spouse. Often their other children have already left home previously or will also be doing so in a couple of years. Unlike the parents of younger ADHD children, these parents are not going to be able to reconnect with their younger children in an effort to try to make things better.

As the marital therapy progresses, the focus can turn to the normal issues of adolescent separation and individuation, but the therapist cannot start at that point as would be the case with other clinical families. The exploration of these issues in marital therapy will confront these historical parenting issues because a spouse may cling to the vulnerability of the ADHD adolescent in order to avoid facing the long-term marital difficulties which will be made more apparent when the child leaves home.

The stages discussed in this chapter identify the multiple levels of interactional dynamics, the explicit roles and attitudes, and the potential dysfunctional processes that may be present for families with ADHD children as they progress through their family life cycle. As such, these stages will help the clinician recognize identifiable patterns, dynamics, and red flags for understanding the family system's experiences. They will also enhance the therapist's clinical assessment and treatment strategies. Certainly, the range of the experiences that we have identified will not always fall within the exact stages that we have defined. Some dynamics may emerge earlier in some families and later in others. In addition, families with multiple ADHD members (parents or children) will display these same patterns but with more drama and greater dysfunctional elements throughout each of these stages. The specific treatment and intervention strategies for ADHD children and adolescents to be presented in the next chapters are intended to interrupt and correct the problematic patterns of behavior as well as the circular struggles that occur in the interactive experiences of the family's system.

6

Developing Therapeutic Interventions for Children with ADHD and Their Families

For many years most of the clinical literature on the treatment of ADHD children was focused primarily on cognitive and behavioral interventions. Yet many controlled outcome studies utilizing cognitive therapeutic approaches display clearly mixed results (Fehlings et al., 1991). A study by Borden and colleagues (1987) reported no significant effects of cognitive training on either academic achievement or behavioral ratings by parents and teachers. Several other studies considered the relationship of cognitive therapies with stimulant medications (Abikoff et al., 1988; Brown et al., 1986, 1988). The Brown et al. (1986) study found that combining cognitive therapy with stimulant medications was no more effective than either approach alone. The Abikoff et al. (1988) study reported no support for the influence of cognitive training on either academic performance or self-esteem enhancement. Some authors (Anastopoulos, 1996; van der Vlugt et al., 1995) have recommended cognitive training programs for the parents of ADHD children. Certainly, other clinical approaches have been discussed in the literature, including a report that brief behavioral interventions reduced some impulsive behaviors (Cocciarella et al., 1995) and that biofeedback reduced some inattentive behaviors (1996).

A SYSTEMIC APPROACH TO ADHD

In this chapter we will describe our work utilizing a family systems orientation and family therapy approaches in working with ADHD children (ranging in ages from infancy to 11 or 12 years) and their families. Working with young children who have ADHD presents the clinician with a variety of challenges and dilemmas. The therapist needs to be able to intervene at a variety of points in the child's family and social systems and to develop a rationale regarding the timing of which members of the family to see, and in which order. Many therapeutic interventions with ADHD children focus solely on interviews with the symptomatic child. We will describe a family intervention approach that we have found to be more effective. We encourage therapists to learn to address and intervene in the roles and dynamics of the broader family system.

Therapists who work primarily in brief and interventive models of psychotherapy, which tend to bypass a patient's history and focus on the goals of alleviating symptoms, will need to recognize the importance of history in understanding and diagnosing ADHD. This does not mean that effective treatment of ADHD needs to be long term, but the historical aspects of evaluation and diagnosis cannot be processed in a hurried manner. Paradoxically, the family therapy methods we use actually reduce the duration of therapy for the ADHD individual because focusing on the family milieu and treating the symptomatic behaviors with a variety of resources (including the family's resources and those of an interdisciplinary network of professionals) facilitate *systemwide*, rather than individually based, changes.

A family systems perspective requires recognition of the broader patterns and dynamics of the family system, from which a variety of interventions can then be selected. The family therapist is never limited to working solely with the source of identified symptoms, whether they exist in a child, a parent, or the marriage. For example, a depressed adult may be understood more accurately when interviewed with her or his marital partner because the symptoms themselves may obscure underlying patterns and/or the partner may bring new data to the interview that would not be available in an individual patient interview. Conduct-disordered adolescents may be understood better when interviewed with their siblings than when interviewed either individually or with their parents. We have reported elsewhere that even in the difficult area of providing psychotherapy with borderline patients, working in the context of the family system clearly reduces treatment time by containing typical symptoms of splitting and projective identification (Everett et al., 1989; Everett & Volgy-Everett, 1998). In other words, the family therapist benefits from being able to choose a variety of points of intervention that are based on both clinical dynamics and the internal resources that can be operationalized within the family itself. The potential range of interventions for ADHD children and their family systems includes the following:

1. The individual child (interview).
2. The individual child (play).
3. The child and parents (interview).
4. The child and parents (play).
5. The parents.
6. The siblings (interview).
7. The siblings (play).
8. The nuclear family system.
9. The marital subsystem.
10. The intergenerational system.

Our model provides a logical sequence of interviews and interventions based on the age of the child and the needs of the family. With most children and adolescents, we begin the therapeutic process, whether or not there is a suggestion of ADHD, by interviewing the *parents without the child*. The parents are the most accurate source of the child's and the family's history. We make every effort to schedule this initial session at a time when both parents can be present. In our first telephone contact we clearly state that we expect both parents to be present and involved. When only one parent shows up for an interview, a major portion of history, as well as reflective parental and marital data, remains unavailable to the therapist. More importantly, the therapist's expectation that both parents attend the initial interview communicates from the start the importance of their mutual roles and involvement in the therapeutic process. We reschedule these initial appointments if one parent calls and says, for example, "My husband is tied up at work, but I would like to come anyway." If we learn from the initiating spouse that her or his partner appears resistant to participating or expresses a preference to not participate, we will offer to call that parent to discuss the importance of his or her presence.

The second session, which is spent with the symptomatic child, occurs in one of several possible formats, depending on the child's age: (1) the child with her or his parents but without the siblings, (2) the child individually in a playroom setting, or (3) the child with her or his sibling(s).

This initial contact with the child is important in developing trust and promoting the child's identification and comfort with the therapist. If scapegoating appears to be present in the family (based on our interview with the parents), as is often the case with ADHD children, we do not schedule an interview with the full family system until we know more about the family's dynamics, especially the roles and attitudes of the sibling(s), and feel confident that we can intervene effectively and control the scapegoating. If the ADHD child is interviewed early on, with family members (parents and/or siblings) who actively attack and scapegoat her or him, the therapist may be unable to deflect the attacks, and repairing the child's consequent distrust of the process may be difficult. We often see older children initially with their siblings, not with their parents. This strategy blurs the focus on the identified child and gives the therapist more power in diverting the scapegoating behaviors, at least within the sibling subsystem. This strategy also provides the therapist with a different perspective on family dynamics as viewed from the siblings' experiences.

As therapy progresses, the therapist may need to conduct interviews with grandparents or other relatives if they have a regular role and ongoing presence in the ADHD child's life. Such interviews are usually most effective when held with as many members of the intergenerational system present as possible. This might include grandparents, aunts and uncles, and the nuclear family members. In addition, as we discussed in Chapters 4 and 5, parental struggles with an ADHD child's behaviors often create difficulties in the parents' marital communication and interactions; in these cases spouses usually benefit greatly from special sessions that focus solely on ways to repair damage in their marriage. Such sessions are most effectively timed following some progress with the specific symptoms and behaviors of the ADHD child. The exception, of course, would be if the spouses are on the verge of separation or divorce.

A TREATMENT MODEL FOR CHILDREN WITH ADHD AND THEIR FAMILIES

Certainly, all families have unique features and dynamics that may dictate a particular pattern of interviews. The model we are presenting (Table 6.1) represents our most effective strategy and most efficient sequencing of interviews, based on our years of clinical practice. There are, of course, areas of necessary modification inherent in any such model. This suggested sequence of interviews is effective if the therapist is beginning an assessment process with an undiagnosed ADHD child or if the child has already been diagnosed and the treatment process is beginning.

Session 1: Parents Only

This initial interview can be the most important in the entire clinical process, for it is here that the therapist creates (or fails to create) a sense of trust and open interaction with the child's parents. Future possibili-

TABLE 6.1. A Model Sequence of Evaluation and Therapy
for ADHD Children and Their Families

Session	Format
1	Parents only; interview
2	Child in play individually or with parent
3	Feedback for parents
4–6	Work with parents
7–9	Work with the child, interview and/or play
10–12	The child and parents in play therapy
12+	Sibling interview
	Nuclear family
	Intergenerational system
	Spouses

ties for positive collaboration will be based on the degree of trust that is forged at this point. Historical documentation of symptomatic patterns are essential to completing the ADHD diagnosis, and parents are usually the primary source of the child's and the family's history. In addition, the parents can provide the therapist with a current description of the child's personal traits and behaviors. Their style of reporting and reflecting also provides the therapist with insight into their own experiences, attitudes, and resources for change.

The initial interview focuses on eliciting details of the child's birth (including the mother's pregnancy) and early development, early health and developmental patterns, social experiences and skills, interaction with siblings and other intergenerational family members, first daycare experiences, initial experiences in kindergarten or first grade, ongoing school experiences and cognitive development, teacher and peer relationships, and present strengths and weaknesses. Information regarding the first 3 years of the child's development should include the parents' early responses to the child and their description of both emotional and behavioral difficulties. We try to gain a clear history of the pregnancy and delivery, including timing of delivery (i.e., Was the child premature or late? By how much?), whether it was natural or induced, type of delivery, the infant's birth weight, APGAR score (if the parents can remember or know what this was), and any early respiratory problems or jaundice. (See Table 6.2.)

We also believe that both the mother's and the father's feelings about the pregnancy are significant. This includes such issues as whether the child was planned or not and what the parents felt when each learned of the pregnancy. It is also important to know whether the infant had a history of very high fevers, seizures, head traumas, or other significant illnesses, and whether there were early hospitaliza-

TABLE 6.2. Components of the Initial Family History Interview with the Parents of an ADHD Child

Family's history

    Early family-of-origin features for both spouses
    Educational histories for both spouses
    Prior marriages and divorces
    Early courtship and marital adjustment
    Prior pregnancies
    Developmental and interactional experiences of earlier children
    School experiences of earlier children
    Parental roles with earlier children
    Specific parental roles with ADHD child
    General coparenting skills and resources
    General marital health, functioning, and boundaries

Child's history

    Mother's and father's prenatal and pregnancy experiences
    Birthing experience
    Early health of the child
    Early developmental patterns
    Early and present social experiences and skills
    Early and present sibling interactions
    Early and present relationships with intergenerational family members
    First daycare experiences
    First experiences in kindergarten and/or first grade
    Ongoing peer and teacher relationships
    Ongoing school experiences and cognitive development
    Cognitive strengths and weaknesses

tions or surgeries. This historical information provides a basis for ruling out the potential for other neurological causes of the child's difficulties. These data are particularly critical in identifying the early warning signs of ADHD symptoms, as well as for noting the responses and resources of the parents at this early stage of treatment.

A child's early physical and emotional responsivity to her or his parents can also be an important indicator of later difficulties. We often hear from parents that their ADHD child was "horrible," "difficult," or "different from the beginning." Indications that the child never liked being held or cuddled, or cried incessantly with colic, or reacted strongly to any stimuli by crying can be markers of early bonding difficulties. However, other parents, particularly those of the inattentive-type child, may tell us that their children were "perfect" during infancy. It is also important to gain information about the child's developmental milestones, such as the age she or he began using words and sentences, began crawling, and started to walk, and especially about any noticeable developmental delays.

During this initial interview, the therapist must also obtain information about the other siblings and their responses to their ADHD sister or brother. Finally, it is imperative that the therapist develop a clinical picture of the family's overall systemic functioning at early and later developmental stages of the child's life. This picture should include such systemic data as a description of the parent's responses to the arrival of each child and the resultant changes in their interactions and boundaries as their parental roles developed.

In addition to gathering data about their children, we also like to ask parents to tell us about how they have fun as a couple, how they use their leisure time individually, and what kinds of activities they enjoy doing as a family unit. We try to determine how much time they actually devote to being together. Significantly, for example, some parents will enthusiastically describe trips and family outings that took place when their children were young, but upon therapist probing will reveal that nothing even close to a pleasant family outing has occurred in many years. It is also important to elicit data that reveal the early structural dynamics in the family. For example, did the father work late hours and/or travel frequently, leaving the mother alone most of the time to care for the ADHD child and their other children? This pattern tends to overwhelm many mothers and deprive the ADHD child and other children of important time with their father. It can also foster excessive dependency on the mother by the children.

In the latter part of this initial interview, we ask the parents about the pluses and minuses of their marriage, delve into issues of privacy and intimacy, and explore communication. The intent here is for an early assessment of the quality of their intimacy and their resources for joint problem solving.

We try to conduct this interview with the parents in a rather casual, engaging, and personal manner as opposed to a more formal history-taking style. The parents need to feel that the therapist is sympathetic and engaged in trying to understand their concerns and struggles. Feeling as if they are being interrogated by a therapist peering at them over a notepad, focused primarily on getting questions answered, does not create an atmosphere conducive to honest, and often painful, disclosure. In our work with families we have learned the value of Nathan Ackerman's (1958) admonishment to family therapists: "Let the live history emerge." The affects expressed by parents, as well as more subtle nonverbal cues, can be as important as the historical data. Since these are usually highly stressed and discouraged individuals by the time they come to a therapist, it is important that in this initial meeting the therapist conveys a sense of warmth and hope. The parents need to feel that their problems are understood, that support is available, and that their sense of despair about their child and their own inadequacies can be alleviated. *Emotionally connecting with parents is the most important element of this initial meeting:* eliciting the detailed history takes second place. If the emotional climate is too intense or volatile, then the therapist must deal with that first and pursue the necessary historical data in an additional session.

Session 2 (3 or 4, If More Sessions Were Needed with the Parents): The Child

In a first meeting with the child, we prefer to see young children under the age of 4 in a play setting with their parents present rather than individually. Often we will ask only the parent who spends the greater amount of time with the child to come to this meeting so that the child does not feel overwhelmed and her or his natural behaviors can still emerge. If both parents are present with a child this young, especially if both parents rarely take the time to play jointly with the child at home, it may create an unnatural environment for the child. In other words, it may be harder to gain an accurate clinical picture of the child's normal behaviors in the play setting if it does not model the interactional patterns in the home. We are aware of the possible concern over excluding the lesser involved parent at this early stage, but for us the more important factor for this particular interview is to gain an accurate impression of the *child's* behaviors. Typically we will have explained this goal carefully to both parents in the prior session. If it seems appropriate for the child and helpful for the therapist, we may schedule a similar interview with the child and the other parent at a later date. Otherwise the excluded parent is assured that his or her involvement in all other family sessions is crucial.

In this initial session the parent and child are simply asked to select toys and play in any way they might normally do at home. The therapist steps back somewhat from the area of play to unobtrusively observe the interaction between the child and the parent. Unlike more formal play therapy, in which the therapist becomes a part of the child's play, the role of the therapist here in the evaluation stage is that of a nonintrusive observer.

Describing our office space and play areas may help illustrate how these interviews are conducted. The physical setting in which the therapist works with an ADHD child is important for several reasons:

1. the active child's need for stimulation, space, and movement.
2. the need to involve the parent(s) in both interviews and play.
3. the need for the therapist to move away and observe the play.

The office of the author (SVE), who works primarily with young children, is separated into distinct interview, play, and activity areas. For therapists like myself who work extensively with young children, the ability to integrate the play area with the interview area can be useful. We believe that an office should be large enough so that there is a clear demarcation between the adult interview space and the child activity space. Some therapists who work with both adults and young children have toys and games scattered throughout their offices, with no clearly identified area for the child except a child-sized chair in a corner. The author's office is rectangular in shape, with a little less than one-third of the space at one end set aside as a work area with desk and bookshelves. The middle one-third of the office is an "adult" interview area with four chairs and a loveseat, lamps, and a table. The other one-third of the office is a play area with a tiled floor, shelves for toys, and a table and four chairs that are child-sized but sturdy example for adults. The toys and games are all ones that can elicit projective, creative play from children. The organization of the office allows the therapist to move into or away from the play area as needed. The chairs have rollers attached and are easily movable so that adults, if they prefer, can roll their chairs into the play area. There is sufficient room for a beanbag chair and pillows so that parents or other members of the family can sit and play on the floor if they wish. For older, more active children, we have a separate playroom (which doubles as a storage area for office materials) equipped with more active toys such as a basketball net, dart games, balls, and other age-appropriate games and items. If the child is 9 years or older, we often use this room for observations and interactions.

These play contexts generally evoke many dynamics and behaviors that are useful in making an evaluation. The therapist can observe the child's level of development in basic areas such as communication and language abilities, social skills, and physical and motor skills. These are also evaluated in terms of the child's expected developmental level. The child's overall range of behaviors, displayed individually or interactively with the parent, are observed especially with respect to possible ADHD indicators such as impulsivity, distractibility, reactivity, frustration intolerance, high activity level, and poor concentration and attention span. The child's relative levels of aggression or passivity are observed, especially toward the parent, both in play and in general interaction.

Our playrooms are equipped with toys that relate to the familial context: dollhouses, with family dollhouse figures; figures representing doctors, nurses, police, firefighters, and other community workers; and stuffed animals and puppets of many kinds. In general, children's toy choices and their manner of play are directly related to their experiences of the world around them. Children use toys as a means of understanding themselves in a variety of contexts. Thus their behaviors in a free-play context provide the therapist with useful indicators of those issues that are most prominent for the child at that time.

The interactive play between the parent and the child provides another set of clinical observations regarding the parent–child relationship. For example: How much does the parent communicate feelings to the child? How interactive is the parent? How reinforcing is the parent? How controlling is the parent with the child? How affectionate, both verbally and physically, is the parent with the child, and vice versa? How patient and gentle is the parent (or the converse)? How does the parent discipline? How consistent and structured is the parent? How nurturant? When the session is over, particularly with very young children, the process of leaving the playroom usually creates a disturbance because the child wants to stay and play. This allows the therapist to see how the parent sets and defines limits when play time is up. Occasionally, this event will erupt into a power struggle and the more difficult behaviors reported by the parents will be acted out in front of the therapist, providing a better grasp of the parents' levels of frustration and discouragement.

Finally, in this session the therapist observes the emotional themes expressed in the child's play. Does the play reveal themes of anger, abandonment, anxieties, or problems with siblings or parents? For example, if parents have resorted to yelling at and hitting the child, the child's play may replicate these experiences. Or the child's play may offer a depiction of a child being scolded and put in time-out. Themes of feeling lonely or rejected, even at this young age, can emerge. These themes, encapsulated in the play experience, provide the therapist with vital information about the emotional difficulties of the child and the behavioral and interactive responses of the parent. If the parent has significant difficulty playing with the child in this session, the therapist may decide to join the child and parent to facilitate more interaction and also to model for the parent what more constructive play with the child might look like. Of course, this must be done in a subtle manner so that the parent is not given the impression that she or he has failed once again. Often, after observing the therapist for a while, the parent gains a better feel for the type of play needed and can take over from the therapist, who then resumes observing the parent–child interaction.

When children are between the ages of 4 and 11, we typically see them individually for at least one session and sometimes for as many as three sessions in a play modality. These play sessions have two primary goals. First, they are designed to establish trust and comfortable interaction between the child and the therapist in a setting where the child experiences minimal anxiety and where she or he can focus solely on toys and play activities. Second, they serve to provide an informal assessment format where, through the therapist's interactions and observations, preliminary clinical hypotheses can be developed with regard to the child's maturity and social and cognitive development. The various issues with younger children identified above can be focused on without the interactional component of the parent's presence. In this experience of play, the therapist must learn to discriminate the cluster of ADHD symptoms that may be interwoven with other difficulties for young children, such as neurological deficits, anxiety disorders, conduct disorders, or depression. These playroom observations and interactions are crucial in aiding the therapist in arriving at a diagnosis and creating a treatment plan. Even if a diagnosis has already been made, these sessions will inform the therapist about the patterns and range of symptoms, as well as provide important information about how the child functions on her or his own.

A 4-year-old boy was referred by his preschool because of his immature behavior and his poor impulse control. The teachers were ready to expel him from the school even though they regarded him as a sweet and lovable child at times. They also recognized that he was probably quite bright. Unfortunately, the boy could go from sharing a toy nicely one minute to hitting a child in the face with it the next moment—which made other mothers worry about their own children's safety. He would cry easily and throw tantrums when he was frustrated or told that he could not do something.

In the play setting the child seemed immediately energized by the sight of the toys. He left his mother's side easily after she brought him into the playroom and excused herself. He immediately began to take things off the shelves in a hurried manner. He would play with something for a few moments and then try something else. When asked questions by the therapist (SVE), he would not answer them unless touched on the arm or shoulder, and then he would give a brief and meaningless answer. Any requests to pick up the toys and return them to the shelves were met with a resounding "No."

His play themes involved being big and tough and everyone being scared of him. He would throw people off rooftops and kick and hit them while yelling, "You're a bad boy." The dollhouse parents yelled at him and told him to go to his room, at which point he said "No" and threw the dollhouse parents down the stairs. He was very distractible and would drop a toy in the middle of a sentence if another toy caught his eye. He paid very little attention to what the therapist was doing unless she entered into the play with him. At those time he would respond within the context of his play but he needed to be the one who controlled what was happening. It was clear that the child was bright; his verbal skills and his complexity of play were excellent when he was able to concentrate on them. However, he could not concentrate long enough to stick with a theme very long and his play interactions were very superficial. This was clearly a child who felt very angry and hurt that others were reprimanding and controlling with him. He conveyed the feeling that no matter what he did, he would be in trouble—which was probably why he did not really try to connect with others unless it suited his own needs.

He was diagnosed with ADHD, hyperactive–impulsive type, and was started on stimulant medication. Following the feedback session with the parents, the therapist asked him to participate in several family therapy sessions; in addition, he took part in play therapy which we offered as a means for him to express his anger and to help him engage in interpersonal contact in a more positive manner. Within a month the parents reported that they, and his teachers, were very pleasantly surprised by the changes he was making; his aggression and impulsivity were considerably improved. They described him as "looking happy for the first time" and as quite manageable with some redirection. The family was able to acknowledge how they had been contributing to his behavioral difficulties by responding to him with anger and punitiveness. The parents were responsive to learning better management and discipline skills, which were experienced by their son as more supportive and loving behaviors.

Session 3 (4 or 5, Depending on the Number of Prior Sessions): Parents' Feedback

Following our initial observations of the ADHD child, we meet with both parents again (without the child present) to share with them our preliminary observations, impressions, and recommendations, trying to point out clearly both their child's strengths and weaknesses. We will also try to relate our observations of the child to aspects of the child's history and/or the child's present behaviors that the parents shared with us in the initial interview. We want to achieve several goals during this feedback session, including:

1. Explain diagnostic impression and information regarding ADHD.
2. Discuss the potential value of referral for an educational assessment and/or testing.
3. Discuss the potential role of medication in treatment and the referral process for medication.

4. Identify other members of the nuclear or extended family system who may have ADHD.
5. Offer a comprehensive plan for treatment: parent sessions, child sessions, consultation with school, consultation with physicians, referral for testing, referral to an educational consultant.

Goal 1

We begin this interview by sharing our diagnostic impressions of the child. If we have sufficient evidence at this point, based on the history, current functioning, and personal observations, to support a diagnosis of ADHD, we share this diagnosis with the parents. If the child has already been diagnosed with ADHD, we relate our observations to the child's symptoms and the behavioral, social, and educational concerns. The therapist's psychoeducational role (discussed in Chapter 4) begins in this session as she or he gives parents additional information on the disorder and comprehensive reasons for the diagnosis.

Goal 2

We discuss the value of an educational assessment and describe the need for testing if none has been conducted. We explain the types of tests necessary and the way we use the data from the tests not only for the diagnosis but also to highlight the child's strengths and weaknesses. We discuss the pros and cons of having the school do the testing versus having the test administered privately. We also identify our network of consultants who can help in various aspects of the evaluation and treatment process.

Goal 3

Next we discuss the medical aspects of the disorder and the potential use of medication—if this seems indicated. We have a couple of brief handouts reviewing medication issues that we give to parents (Miller, 1994). Because the topic of medicating a young child can be quite intimidating and frightening for parents, we introduce the topic tentatively and carefully, putting off decisions regarding medication until after testing is completed and further interaction with the child and the parents has occurred. We are careful not to step into the role of the physician, who is the proper professional to discuss with the parents the appropriate type of medication, dosage levels, and potential side effects, and the like. Parents typically ask about waiting several years or until the child has started grade school to reevaluate for medication. We give the parents an opportunity to verbalize their concerns and to then try to alleviate their fears and misgivings about the use of medication. The therapist needs to be aware that this issue of medication can be very difficult if the child is five years or younger; parents tend to experience a much higher level of protectiveness with their preschool children and may be more resistant to the suggestion of medication at these early ages. The therapist must be prepared to listen attentively to and understand these parental concerns in a nonjudgmental manner, even if it is quite clear that medication would benefit a hyperactive–impulsive ADHD child immediately. We try to present the role of medication in the broader picture of building self-esteem rather than simply controlling behavior. We also often tell them about a variety of other case situations in which medication has been beneficial.

Goal 4

Our next goal is to learn more about the possible existence of ADHD elsewhere in the family system or in the parents' families of origin. Often by this point in the interview one parent has already volunteered that she or he had similar symptoms as a child (and still has them, in most cases), or one spouse points out that the symptom description seems to apply to the partner. We also ask about each parent's families of origin, particularly in terms of parents or siblings having had similar difficulties in school. While we are discussing these issues, we typically ask about histories of depression, serious emotional difficulties, or substance abuse in the family. If one of the parents believes that she or he may also have ADHD, we broaden our discussion to include information about adult ADHD and the possibility of their own need for diagnosis and treatment (see Chapter 8). This is an important clinical window for identifying undiagnosed ADHD in a parent or another child because the relevant information emerges naturally from the discussion and concerns regarding their child, who is unmistakably troubled. We have found the process of identifying ADHD to be much easier in this context than in the context of working with an undiagnosed ADHD adult in either individual or marital therapy. As we noted previously, the failure to recognize ADHD in parents, or elsewhere in the family's system, can sabotage not only the therapist's efforts to improve parent–child relations but also other interventions directed at facilitating healthier interactions among family members.

Goal 5

Finally, we develop an overall treatment plan which, of course, varies with the age of the child and the unique family situation. Even though firm decisions, particularly regarding testing or medication, need not be finalized in this session, the next steps in the evaluation and treatment process need to be made clear for the parents by the end of this session. If we are going to ask parents to consult with our medical or educational colleagues, we will formalize that plan at this point.

Sessions 4–6 (Possibly 6–8): Parental Sessions

Most parents who bring their child to therapy, either on their own or by referral from a school or physician, have experienced considerable prior struggles and frustrations with the child's behaviors and functioning. We have found that the more effective initial interventions occur with the parents, not with the ADHD child. Even parents who express a sense of relief that someone else is in charge of evaluating—and perhaps finally explaining—their child's struggles will need assistance in undoing entrenched patterns and gaining a sense of control in the family. These sessions are therefore designed specifically for the parents and focus on giving them more detailed psychoeducational information regarding ADHD, discussing how it affects their family's functioning on many levels, and teaching them more effective child management skills. Given the parents' high levels of frustration and often their feelings of helplessness, and even hopelessness, they should be encouraged to implement these new skills immediately; often significant positive effects become apparent within 2 to 4 weeks. The following goals shape the content and number of these parental sessions:

1. Discuss the impact of ADHD on the entire family system in greater detail.
2. Provide child management training.
3. Identify any comorbid symptoms.
4. Reduce overall stress as quickly as possible through structural and/or behavioral parental interventions.
5. Continue to assess the general resources and strengths of the parents as well as their patterns of marital communication and interaction.
6. Schedule consultation with a child psychiatrist or other physician to discuss medication issues.

7. Schedule interviews with psychometrist and/or educational consultant.

(Depending on the dynamics of the case, these goals may be postponed until after the therapy process has begun and discussion with the school has occurred.)

Goal 1

The initial goal is to help the parents understand the specific etiology and nature of the disorder and to give them the opportunity to ask questions, reveal their fears, and reflect on how the disorder has influenced their parenting roles and family experiences. We give parents a variety of handouts and a list of reading resources (see Appendix 6.1). If the parents seem interested, we mention the parent support groups that are sponsored by the CHADD organization in our community. We have learned that an individual's first impressions about a support group are often lasting. Thus there is no benefit in pushing parents toward these support groups prematurely. Many parents need time to understand and integrate the ADHD issues privately before they approach a support group. Some parents are embarrassed about their child's diagnosis and what it represents in terms of their parenting frustrations and struggles. If the parents are anxious about this recommendation, we tell them about these opportunities and suggest that they consider participating at a later date.

Goal 2

The practical focus of these three sessions is to provide the parents with new skills—easily learned and readily applied—to aid them in their everyday tasks of parental management. Depending on the age of the child, we may focus on issues of family structure (hierarchy, boundaries, alliances, etc.), behavioral management, and/or communication and support between spouses and within the family. If the child is under age 9, often our initial task is to teach the parents specific behavior management skills. We believe that appropriate time-outs are the most effective discipline technique for ADHD children from the ages of 3 to about 9 years. The standard recommendation of 1 minute for every year of age is not effective with ADHD children. We categorize three types of time-out settings, with recommended times for each: (1) the child's bedroom (with the door closed), with the time-out ranging from no less than 15 minutes to no more than 45 minutes; (2) a chair in an isolated and quiet part of the home, with the time-out ranging from 5 minutes up to the age of 5 to 10 minutes for ages 6 and 7 (not recommended for children older than 7); or (3) a specified time-out room, such as the laundry room or a bathroom, with the time-out ranging from 5 to 10 minutes, depending on the age and offense. This system of time-out settings is important with ADHD children because of the need to dramatically reduce the stimulation they receive from other family members and the environment.

We then describe the types of time-outs that are appropriate for differing behaviors. (These methods may not be very different from those used with children with other behavioral disorders.) We are very specific regarding recommended amounts of time appropriate for differing ages and behaviors, the conditions to impose, and how to select the proper setting. For ADHD children, a time-out may need to cover the actual period when the child is in a calming-down phase. This means that the time-out begins only when the child is less reactive, that the timer is reset if the reactions recur at any point, and that an additional 5 minutes is added each time the child leaves the time-out setting. Due to their difficulties with short-term memory, time-outs for ADHD children need to be initiated *immediately* after the inappropriate behavior. If the parents wait, even a few minutes, the intervention may have very little benefit. Time-outs may also need to be somewhat longer for ADHD children because they require more time to gain control of their reactive behaviors.

We teach parents the basic use of rewards, token systems, and other behavioral methods, stressing the importance of how consistency, structure, and predictability can help reduce the frequency of difficult behaviors related to anxiety. We help parents understand that if they want to change behaviors, rewarding ADHD children is far more powerful than punishing them. Physical punishment in particular can exacerbate an ADHD child's volatility and reactivity. Thus we caution parents that this method only serves to increase stimulation and punitiveness, to which the child is unusually sensitive. We also teach the parents that yelling and belligerent interactions may also serve only to amplify the symptoms and difficulties, and we suggest ways to help them control their own impulses and reduce the intensity of their own reactions. These sessions offer parents an alternative to hitting or yelling at their ADHD child by providing them with the tools for which they have been desperately searching. Parents often tell us, "I've tried *everything* and nothing works"; their discouragement, which is palpable in the room, has often been an unwanted companion for many years.

We try to help parents understand that the many methods they have tried without positive results failed because they were not consistently and clearly enforced. Most parents move quickly from method to method in their desperation to find a way to change things; when one method does not immediately work, it is abandoned and replaced with another. Reflection on their application of a method simply does not occur in these highly stressed conditions. Some parents have very limited parenting skills or their degree of emotional overload has prevented them from accessing the skills and resources they already possess. When the parents begin to apply the new techniques we teach them in a consistent manner, they find that their ADHD child quickly becomes more manageable and much more pleasant to be around. Thanks to the positive results they experience early in the treatment process, the parents quickly begin to feel a restored confidence in their parenting. Now a productive and refreshing cycle is finally in place: increasingly pleasant interactions occur between the parents and their ADHD child because the parents are beginning to feel effective and capable; concurrently, the child is feeling not only more in control of her or his impulses but also more accepted and appreciated within the family.

If the therapist is clear and realistic in teaching appropriate management skills, most parents will develop more positive expectations and their efforts will produce a new level of efficacy. The emphasis on providing the child with structure, predictability, consistency, and reduction of parental reactivity is extremely important. Many parents struggle with emotional difficulties that impede their ability to assess situations by using all of their resources. These difficulties include pervasive personal discouragement and even grief over having an ADHD child. Once the therapist can identify these issues and bring them out into the open, the parents experience a sense of relief and unburdening that frees them to begin to use more effective and practical skills.

Goal 3

As we are working with the parents, we also look for any comorbid symptoms in the ADHD child, which generally begin to appear during the grade school years. We are careful to look for signs of anxiety, depression, oppositional defiant disorder, or conduct disorders. It is quite common for an ADHD child to develop additional emotional difficulties as a result of the behavioral and interactional problems that are a part of the symptom cluster for ADHD. The types of comorbid problem areas that emerge in a particular child depend on many factors, including the basic temperament of the child, the personalities of the parents and their history of parenting, the home environment, school experiences, unrelated traumatic events, relationships with extended family members, and health history. Whatever the comorbid pattern, it is important for the therapist to recognize that additional symptoms can become imbedded in the behaviors of the ADHD child and in the perceptions and responses of family members toward that child. In other words, the comorbid symptoms often become as central to the family's interactions and functioning as the ADHD symptoms.

The literature certainly indicates that most ADHD children develop comorbid dysfunctional patterns such as depression, anxiety, oppositional defiant disorder, and even conduct disorders. For example, although oppositional defiant disorder is often associated more with adolescent behaviors, it may appear as early as ages 3 or 4. This child opposes all attempts to control or manage her or his behavior and creates power struggles over the simplest requests. In adolescence these oppositional behaviors take the form of reactivity, argumentativeness, uncooperativeness, opposing parental rules, and often a need for control. Younger ADHD children with oppositional defiant disorder fight and argue over any instruction that is contrary to their preference. They may also call the parent derogatory names and create embarrassing scenes in public places if their demands are not immediately met. These children often intimidate their parents with their volatile behaviors, making them feel immobilized and unable to control and manage these situations.

The parents of a 7-year-old boy tearfully told one of the authors (SVE) that she was at wit's end with her child. She reported that he stubbornly refused to do even minor tasks such as dress or eat breakfast. He would erupt into a rage at the slightest provocation and scream obscenities at her even in public. Any attempts to apply consequences only intensified his rage, and the mother was completely unable to manage him. Although the school reported fewer displays of rage, in the home his temper and refusal to cooperate with anyone often controlled the interactions of the entire family. He would not leave his mother's side except to go to school and was quite immature and anxious if she was not with him. His anxiety led him to want to sleep with his mother anytime his father was away and to want to control her every move to the extent that she could not be out of his sight. Due to the parent's associated marital problems, it had become increasingly difficult for them to manage his problem behaviors jointly. The brunt of the parenting was left to the mother, who also had three other children to raise. By now she was depressed, discouraged, exhausted, and angry.

This child certainly had a number of apparent emotional difficulties, such as depression and anxiety, as well as conduct problems. However, following the initial interview with the parents and a review of the history, it became clear that there was an underlying disorder of ADHD. The testing confirmed the ADHD symptoms and also indicated that he was a bright child. He was placed on both an antidepressant and a stimulant medication. The following sessions were divided between time with the parents regarding management issues and joint sessions with the child and the parents. Later the entire family was seen, with all four children present.

The parents learned how they were contributing to his conduct problems by their inconsistent and impotent responses to his rages. After teaching them some behavioral management skills, the therapist shifted focus to their marital issues. In those sessions the parents were able to express and gain closure on their past discouragements and hurt feelings with one another. They also agreed to set aside some time for their own relationship. Gradually they began to work jointly with the child in a much more helpful way. Many of the child's difficult behaviors began to subside. They reported that he appeared to be more self-reliant, less anxious (anxiety triggered many of his rage reactions), and more cooperative. They also reported that they felt more successful and in touch with the needs of their other three children. In this case the medications helped give the child some control over his own moods and behaviors. However, the medications alone would not have been sufficient to create the improvements that occurred. It was also essential that the parents learned better parenting skills and repaired the damage in their own relationship.

Goal 4

The primary goal at this early stage in the therapeutic process is to reduce, as quickly as possible, the overall stress and chaos that many ADHD families experience. In addition to issues of behavioral management, we therefore also discuss the parents' roles and relationship with the other children and their behaviors in the family, especially relationships with their ADHD sibling. These issues often present an opportunity to teach the parents about the hierarchy, structure, and boundary patterns present in their family. These structural concerns are pursued clinically in the family sessions when all of the children are present. Additional clinical interventions involve deflecting some of the negative focus away from the scapegoated ADHD child and enhancing the parents' time and relationships with the other siblings.

Goal 5

Throughout these interviews, we are assessing the strengths and resources of the parents, both individually and as a couple. We are concerned about their levels of frustration and anger, as well as their potential for scapegoating or abusing the ADHD child. We are also concerned about the health of their marriage, their level of intimacy, and their degree of mutual communication. In ADHD families the parents' marital boundaries, which are sorely needed to protect their own relationship, are often weak and diffuse. Therefore, much of the clinical work with the couple should be focused on defining and strengthening their boundaries, removing their excessive focus on parenting the ADHD child, and improving their levels of intimacy and communication.

In these early interviews, the therapist also needs to assess the available emotional resources of the parents in order to facilitate more realistic treatment planning. The therapist needs to accurately judge what the parents are capable of learning and doing so that the therapy itself does not create another experience of failure for them. *We often tell parents that they are the real therapists for their child,* and that they will need to learn the skills to take over and continue when the therapy process ends. We also believe that it is important to limit the duration of our therapeutic relationship with an ADHD child to as brief a period as possible. *Extended, long-term therapy with ADHD children is usually unnecessary if the family, which is the focus of treatment, can make broader systemic changes.* Such long-term therapy only serves to reinforce the child's self-perception of being "damaged." This is why, especially for younger ADHD children, we involve the parents from the very beginning and make every effort to initiate family sessions as soon as possible so that treatment is shared by the whole family and is not focused exclusively on the ADHD child. Therefore, many of these initial sessions are designed with the educational purpose of providing parents with the knowledge and skills to become advocates for their ADHD child and to create a healthier family environment for all of their children.

Goal 6

With families where we are relatively certain about the appropriateness of the ADHD diagnosis (particularly when we are working with hyperactive–impulsive ADHD children of this age), we will raise the issues of utilizing stimulant medications with the parents even before testing has been completed. If parents are cautious and uncertain about the effects of medication and fearful of making the decision to medicate their child, we arrange for them to meet briefly with one of our consulting physicians. In our own practices, we work closely with a child psychiatrist, so we ask him to stop in for a few minutes during one of our sessions with the parents to answer their questions and provide them with medical information. The parents may also be referred to another physician if they prefer to work with their child's pediatrician or if their medical insurance requires such consultation. In these cases we call the physician's office and leave a message in the presence of the parents so that they can hear the referral being made. Often a trusted family pediatrician or physician can alleviate parents' apprehensions regarding medications and help them with the emotional decision to medicate their child.

Goal 7

At the conclusion of these initial sessions with the parents, we usually have a firm evaluation and treatment plan in place (see Table 6.3). This includes a plan for when and by whom the child will be tested and an appointment to meet together again to review the testing data. As part of this treatment plan the therapist should be prepared to say who will be seen, in what order, and for approximately how long, and to explain the specific goals of each interview. If medication is recommended, the choice of physician should be decided upon, and a time frame for the assessment to take place should be established. The parents are given ample time to ask questions, make comments, or discuss issues related to the recommendations.

Sessions 7–9+: The Child

The next stage of the ongoing treatment is to work with the ADHD child individually in a play setting. The clinical goals are to address the child's emotional, behavioral, and interactional issues. Since most children at this age are not insight-oriented, individual play therapy sessions allow the therapist to observe the child and begin teaching appropriate behaviors and create better executive functioning abilities for the child. This is accomplished by allowing the child to select play objects and then intervening to reinforce her or his quality of play, with the goal of increasing self-esteem and appropriate self-manage-

---

TABLE 6.3. The Components of an Initial Treatment Plan for Young ADHD Children and Their Families

1. Arrange for psychoeducational testing, specifying when and by whom.
2. Schedule a time to review testing data with the parents.
3. Discuss when and how to pursue medical consultation.
4. Schedule the next parent sessions.
5. Specify the timing of the child play sessions.
6. Specify the timing of the future family therapy sessions.
7. Consider the need for future marital and/or intergenerational sessions.
8. Consider the need for consultation with an educational consultant.

ment. Play is the medium used to enhance self-reflection and to rehearse appropriate behavior with others in their environment. A child may play with family figures in a dollhouse, for example, to replicate patterns of interaction in his or her own family that may dramatize frustrations and failures. The therapist helps the child, using the dollhouse figures, to learn more satisfactory behaviors with family members. When a new positive outcome emerges in the play, this new outcome helps the child understand that these new behaviors can be effective. The use of play allows the child to decrease her or his anxiety in parent–child and social interactions, and provides a model for more positive relationships. (For readers who are less familiar with approaches to play therapy, we recommend attending workshops offered by experienced play therapists to develop these skills.)

We devote only a few sessions to individual therapy with younger ADHD children so that the focus of treatment can be returned to the parent–child relationship. The exact number of sessions needed is dependent on a variety of factors related to the child, parent, and family dynamics. The therapist needs to be flexible in moving between individual play with the child, to parent–child interaction and play, and then to broader family sessions. It has been our experience that when all evaluation and treatment plans are put into effect—testing, medication, improving the school environment, improving parenting behaviors, stabilizing the family environment, and providing emotional assistance—progress occurs quite rapidly. In fact, many parents, having struggled for years with their ADHD child, will often express surprise and amazement at the significant behavioral changes that occur in a short period of time.

Sessions 10+: Parents and Child in Play Therapy

As noted above, it is important to move as quickly as possible to these parent–child interactional sessions that include only the ADHD child; the siblings will be invited to attend the following family therapy sessions. However, these parent–child sessions must be timed carefully so that they occur only after significant progress has been made. It can be a poignant experience for the ADHD child to play with her or his parents without being reprimanded or yelled at, without fighting or being pressured, and where laughter and enjoyment of each other fill the room. The therapist's role in these sessions is to (1) model effective parenting techniques, (2) reinforce the parents' efforts to achieve a level of joint communication and management that fosters executive functioning in their child, and (3) facilitate increased levels of positive interaction among parents and child. These goals can be accomplished in a variety of ways. For example, the therapist might ask the child to select an area of play, such as building blocks or the dollhouse, and then ask the parents to join in the activity. As the three interact, the therapist observes the parents' exchange with each other and their responses to the child and intervenes, if necessary, to steer their interactions in a direction that reinforces cooperative behaviors and enhances self-esteem. As the session proceeds, the parents are encouraged to use their own resources to guide the interaction and, at the conclusion of the session, to assume a clear parental role by bringing an end to the play, putting away the toys, and preparing to leave. The therapist assists the parents, if necessary, in dealing supportively with the child's potential resistance to stopping play. The therapist may employ a variety of psychotherapeutic games for the family. These games are interactive and encourage family members to discuss feelings, activities, and experiences together. The play associated with these games increases emotional sensitivity among family members in a context that is fun and playful.

Sessions 12+: Family Therapy Sessions

After some progress has been made in parent management skills, family therapy sessions are scheduled that include the parents, the ADHD child, the siblings, and any live-in relatives or potential caretakers. The greatest potential for therapeutic change regarding the family's perceptions of, and reactions to, the child's ADHD symptoms lies in these family sessions. We usually conduct family therapy sessions when the ADHD child is at least 4 years of age or older. (This may not be a comfortable approach for those therapists unaccustomed to working with young children; of course, the more experienced the therapist is in this area the more effective will be the therapeutic outcome.)

Although these family therapy sessions can become the primary setting for clinical change, that will be the case only when they have been preceded by preparatory stages of evaluation and diagnosis, parent education, and interaction with the child in play therapy. These initial clinical interventions provide the foundation for later change by clearly identifying the problem areas, providing the parents with better tools for managing all of their children's behaviors, and focusing the family's efforts on explicitly attainable goals. *If these family sessions were conducted from the onset, before this foundation was properly laid, the chaos and frustrations of all of the family members would simply be replicated, often unmanageably, in the therapist's office.* Similarly, if the siblings are involved in the therapy process too early, their habitual scapegoating will be used predictably to attack the ADHD sibling and disrupt any progress that has been made. The therapist can rely on the early parent education and child play sessions to establish some progress and demonstrate the potential for change so that the siblings' experiences at home will already have been challenged either by the improvements they may witness in their ADHD sibling (particularly if she or he has been medicated successfully) or by their parents' improved ways of relating and parenting.

Family therapists need to select a therapeutic role carefully with regard to their level of involvement and style of intervention. An overly passive stance with chaotic families only exacerbates their turmoil. But while clear direction and structure is needed, that, too, can be overdone. Intervening in an overly active or controlling manner with these families only gets in the way of family members learning to engage and act on their own with new resources. We have found that when the therapist provides gentle direction and prodding, family members will learn to use their own resources nearly 80% of the time.

However, the therapist will need to take a more directive role temporarily with those ADHD families who remain somewhat chaotic even at this later stage in order to define limits and establish more structure for the interactions. For example, in some cases it may be necessary for the therapist to align with the parents and structure the session so that they are physically seated next to one another without a child between them. This helps to define the parents' roles and power in the system in a symbolic manner. In other situations the therapist might need to engage the siblings more directly in order to gain their attention, block their scapegoating of the ADHD sibling, and model for the parents a new management role. At times, particularly in more chaotic family systems, the therapist might be tempted to align with, and seek to protect, the ADHD child. Clinically there is little to be gained by such an intervention because the therapist cannot continue that role with the family on the way home from the therapy session. The family needs to find their own resources to cease the scapegoating and the parents need to gain the strength to manage the family's interactions better.

The specific goals of these family therapy sessions vary according to the dynamics of each family system and the age of the ADHD child. However, there are several central goals that appear to be common with most ADHD families:

1. Block and extinguish the patterns of scapegoating.
2. Reinforce and empower the parents' newly defined roles in the family.
3. Define and strengthen the parents' boundaries.

4. Stabilize and enhance the marital relationship.
5. Define and adjust intergenerational boundaries, if necessary.

Goal 1

Both parents and siblings engage in the process of scapegoating the ADHD child. By the start of these family therapy sessions the parents ideally have gained some new skills in parenting so that their frustrations have diminished somewhat and they are willing to learn and try new ways of interacting. Occasionally scapegoating of the ADHD child reappears simply because it has been embedded emotionally in the family's interactions for many years. If the therapist intervenes quickly at the first signs of scapegoating, it should dissipate quickly. Interventions directed at blocking, diffusing, and/or redirecting the scapegoating dynamics are effective. At this stage, the scapegoating comes more from the siblings, who have not had the benefit of the earlier parent–child interaction and education sessions.

Here the therapist's strategy is to enlist the new resources of the parents to help block the scapegoating attacks by siblings. Utilizing the parents' resources to reshape the family's emotional experience becomes a powerful clinical intervention. If the siblings are resistant to the parents' efforts to interrupt the scapegoating cycle, the therapist simply reinforces the parents' new role in the family or occasionally models behaviors that block the destructive interactions. For example, the therapist might interrupt a sibling's attack by engaging a parent or another sibling in a conversation about an unrelated theme. In chaotic families, structural interventions that reshape the alliances and roles within the family are effective. In this case, the attacking sibling may be asked to sit next to the therapist, next to the ADHD child, or next to the more powerful parent, thereby challenging her or his power and pattern of attacking. If necessary, the therapist might assume a role as a commentator on the progress the family has made and as an interpreter of the ADHD child's particular challenges and difficulties. This leads to the second major goal.

Goal 2

No matter how many new skills and resources the parents have learned by this stage, the development of lasting positive changes for the family will be dependent upon their learning to access and act on their own resources. As we indicated above, it is important for the therapist to facilitate this process and allow the parents' resources to emerge in this context with their children present. If progress has been made in the early stages of the treatment sequence, the parents' specific roles in relation to the ADHD child and the non-ADHD siblings can be enhanced and empowered in a minimum of family sessions. If the progress is slower and the scapegoating continues, the therapist may need to take a more active role, as described, to block the scapegoating and model more effective roles for the parents.

Structural family interventions can be quite helpful at this point in the process (Minuchin, 1974; Minuchin & Fishman, 1981; Nichols & Everett, 1987). Useful structural interventions at this time include the following:

• The therapist asks the parents to sit side by side during the interview to block an intrusive or controlling child who insists on sitting between them. This move symbolically demonstrates, both for the parents themselves and for their children, clearer parental boundaries and roles, and increases the parents' sense of control in the family.

• The scapegoated ADHD child is asked to sit next to the therapist for part of a session to enhance her or his role. This move will symbolically attribute additional status to the child and may block scapegoating until the parents can gain more control. We will often ask the ADHD child, who is now seated next to us, to be a "consultant" and help us understand how the family works or what roles Mom and Dad play in the family. We would never place the ADHD child between the parents because we are trying to define and protect their boundaries, while at the same normalizing and strengthening the role of the ADHD child in the family's overall interactions.

• A particularly resistant and angry non-ADHD sibling may be asked to sit next to the therapist as a "consultant." This helps the therapist gain some control over the sibling's anger and interruptions in the session and often diffuses her or his attacks on the ADHD sibling or the parents by suddenly redefining her or his role in the family.

Goal 3

In order to accomplish the above goal of empowering the parents' role in the family, their ineffective or absent boundaries must be addressed. Spouses in ADHD families have often become quite child-focused, allowing the behaviors of their children, particularly the ADHD child, to intrude into all their interactions and decision making. The establishment of clear and firm boundaries has positive implications for both parental and marital dynamics. These boundaries must be drawn to allow the parents a protective space in which they can develop a coparenting relationship and learn to work as a team. This is a typical struggle for most parents in ADHD families.

The development of these boundaries must occur in the experiential context of the family's interaction in these family therapy sessions. Boundary concepts can be discussed abstractly in separate sessions with parents, but the creation of the boundaries themselves must evolve from the parents' actual interactional behaviors in the system. Here the therapist can help parents define these boundaries by removing an intrusive child from between them; by having the parents sit together—to signify their joint authority—and somewhat separate from the rest of the family—to highlight an appropriate degree of distance; or by modeling effective boundary-setting behaviors with the children. Several additional family sessions may be necessary to reinforce and stabilize these new boundary patterns at home. However, many parents tells us that once they learned to recognize and define their boundaries, they became more confident, were able to assume more control at home, and now recognized when the children were attempting to sabotage their roles and get in between them. This process of successfully defining parent–child boundaries should also have an observable positive impact on the parents' marital relationship.

Goal 4

Marital interactions for the parents of young ADHD children may have become problematic, but during this early period of living with ADHD children they are not as distant or conflicted as the parents of undiagnosed ADHD adolescents (which we will discuss further in the next chapter). Part of this family therapy stage of treatment involves conducting several sessions with the parents as a marital couple. These sessions may need to be scheduled intermittently, alternating with the family sessions, when the process of defining boundaries is blocked due to underlying marital conflict or distance. Unless one of the spouses is considering divorce, usually only a few marital sessions are needed to help them clarify and revive their commitment to one another and to recognize the benefit to them as a couple of gaining more control in their family. In other words, in addition to improving their parenting, the parents also benefit from changes that enhance their own personal levels of closeness and intimacy. Most parents of ADHD children report having lost all sense of the emotional connectedness that characterized their early romantic involvement with one another. However, once they begin to feel more confident as parents, their prior experiences of attraction and bonding can often be rediscovered and renewed.

Goal 5

Grandparents and other family-of-origin members may play intrusive roles that exacerbate the parenting problems and school failures of an ADHD child in the family. We have worked with many families where a well-meaning grandparent, uncle, or aunt has openly accused both parents of inadequate parenting and blamed them for the undiagnosed child's problematic behaviors and school failures. Even after a diagnosis has been confirmed, some of these family-of-origin members may persist in their unrelenting attacks on the parents and even the ADHD child.

These dynamics need to be identified and controlled therapeutically as quickly as possible. In some cases the intervention may involve simply helping the parents create some emotional distance from these intrusive criticisms, particularly if the relatives reside some distance away. However, we also believe that it is important for families to maintain and nurture their intergenerational ties and resources, so we are careful to offer other ways of controlling or diffusing these intergenerational intrusions. For example, we often offer to invite these family-of-origin members, typically grandparents, to attend a session with the parents. (We suggest that therapists who have not conducted family-of-origin therapy or consultation sessions refer to Framo, 1992.) If these family members live nearby or are planning a trip to visit soon, we will schedule a consultation session with both parents and the visiting grandparents but not the children. We may give the grandparents the same diagnostic information that we reviewed with the parents, discuss the role of the testing, the test results, and the use of stimulant medications. We describe the progress that we have made and the positive changes that everyone has observed in the ADHD child and in the family a whole. The grandparents may ask questions, but usually this one session is sufficient to diffuse their critical roles. In some cases, we may help their adult child discuss with them the type of relationship they need now, as well as what would benefit the ADHD grandchild. Sometimes the parent wishes to set a firmer boundary with the grandparents, but other times the parent asks for involvement of a more supportive nature.

Grandparents and other relatives typically express their appreciation when we include them in the therapy process. On a few occasions we have conducted telephone interviews with the grandparents, using the speaker phone with the parents present, with similar helpful effects. We find these intergenerational sessions to be most productive when they are scheduled after considerable improvements have been made. However, they can occur earlier in the clinical sequence if the family-of-origin members are arriving spontaneously for a visit or if they live near the parents and play a more active everyday role in the family.

The actual number of the family therapy sessions may vary from two to eight, depending on the dynamics that need to be addressed, the success in reducing the ADHD child's problematic symptoms, and the success in reshaping the parenting roles. We cannot overemphasize the value of incorporating family therapy sessions in working with ADHD children. Accomplishing lasting clinical changes for the child and the family cannot happen by focusing solely on the child. Many early steps toward progress, such as medication or school interventions, can be negated easily and quickly when the treatment is terminated prematurely, that is, before the parents, siblings, and even relatives have improved their interactions and quality of life together.

The clinical sequence that we have described progresses from assessment and/or diagnosis to parent education/therapy to family therapy sessions involving the ADHD child and the other siblings. The timing of this sequence allows the therapist to focus initially on the ADHD symptoms and their effects on the family's interaction. The therapist then directs interventions toward aiding the parents in developing a better understanding of their child's ADHD and learning more effective management skills that will benefit the parenting of all their children. The potential use of stimulant medication is important to consider at these stages as an additional aid for the ADHD child. Progress in these areas allows the therapist to focus next, and more effectively, on the interaction of the entire family system, which may also include marital and intergenerational issues. The sequence of this overall model is based on our clinical experiences and, of course, our own clinical styles. We certainly believe that other approaches and clinical interventions can be successful with ADHD families. However, we hope that the observations we have noted at each stage in the model will provide the therapist with a better picture of what to look for and how to develop effective intervention strategies. In the next chapter we will present a similar clinical sequence for working with ADHD adolescents and their families.

APPENDIX 6.1. READING RESOURCES AND SUPPORT ORGANIZATIONS FOR FAMILY MEMBERS

For Parents

Barkley, R. (1995). *Taking charge of ADHD.* New York: Guilford Press.

Cohen, M. (1997). *The attention zone.* New York: Brunner/Mazel.

Diller, L. (1998). *Running on ritalin: A physician reflects on children, society, and performance in a pill.* New York: Bantam

Dornbush, M., & Pruitt, S. (1995). *Teaching the tiger: A handbook for individuals involved in the education of students with attention deficit disorders, Tourette syndrome or obsessive–compulsive disorder.* Durate, CA: Hope Press.

Kennedy, P., Terdal, L., & Fusetti, L. (1993). *The hyperactive child book.* New York: St. Martin's Press.

Kilcarr, P., & Quinn, P. (1997). *Voices from fatherhood—Fathers, sons and ADHD.* New York: Brunner/Mazel.

McCarney, S., & Johnson, N. (1995). *The parent's guide to early childhood attention deficit disorders intervention manual.* Columbia, MO: Hawthorne Educational Services.

Weiss, L. (1994). *The attention deficit disorder in adults workbook.* Dallas: Taylor Publishing.

For Children

Ingersoll, B. (1995). *Distant drums, different drummers.* Bethesda, MD: Cape Publishing.

Moss, D. (1989). *SHELLEY the hyperactive turtle.* Rockville, MD: Woodbine House.

Quinn, P., & Stern, J. (1992). *Putting on the brakes.* New York: Magination Press.

Quinn, P., & Stern, J. (1993). *Putting on the brakes activity book.* New York: Magination Press.

For Adolescents

Gordon, M. (1992). *I would if I could: A teenager's guide to ADHD/hyperactivity.* New York: GSI Publications.

Nadeau, K. (1994). *Survival guide for college students with ADD or LD.* New York: Brunner/Mazel.

Quinn, P. (1995). *Adolescents and ADD: Gaining the advantage.* New York: Brunner/Mazel.

Quinn, P. (1994). *ADD and the college student.* New York: Brunner/Mazel.

For Adults

Hallowell, E., & Ratey, J. (1994). *Driven to distraction.* New York: Pantheon.

Hallowell, E., & Ratey, J. (1994). *Answers to distraction.* New York: Pantheon.

Hartmann, T. (1993). *ADD: A different perception.* Penn Valley, CA: Underwood.

Kelly, K., & Ramundo, P. (1993). *You mean I'm not lazy, stupid or crazy?!* New York: Scribner.

Nadeau, K. (1996). *Adventures in fast forward: Life, love, and work for the ADD adult.* New York: Brunner/Mazel.

Nadeau, K. (1997). *ADD in the workplace: Choices, changes, and challenges.* New York: Brunner/Mazel.

Organizations and Resources

Children and Adults with Attention Deficit Disorders (CHADD)
National Conference and Quarterly Magazine
499 NW 70th Avenue, Suite 101
Plantation, Florida 33317
http://www.chadd.org/

ADD WareHouse
A catalog of books, products and other resources
300 NW 70th Avenue, Suite 102
Plantation, Florida 33317
1-800-233-9273

7

Developing Therapeutic Interventions for Adolescents with ADHD and Their Families

The beginning of adolescence as a specific developmental period cannot always be identified precisely. The onset of puberty is seen as one line of demarcation, but puberty is a measure of physiological, not emotional, development. Some youngsters mature physically, but remain quite immature emotionally. Many ADHD adolescents can be up to 2 years behind others same-age peers in their level of social maturity and their ability to make sound decisions. Some ADHD adolescents are a year or more behind when they should be in school and thus still in grade school at age 13; obviously, typical adolescent issues arise somewhat later for these children than for their peers. For others, these same issues arise, but they are not ready to handle them.

Nevertheless, there are prominent features that differentiate both the symptoms of and the treatment program for ADHD adolescents from the symptoms and treatment of ADHD children. Compared to children, adolescents may experience greater levels of personal discouragement and frustration, heightened awareness of their "differentness" and of a divide that isolates them from siblings and peers, and less self-confidence and lower self-esteem. Some will report greater levels of distractions and consequent confusion in the more complex settings of middle and high school, more demanding academic challenges, and higher risks of school failure. Others experience greater risks of legal consequences as a result of their hyperactive–impulsive behaviors, higher levels of parental frustration and intolerance, and greater risks for family violence. Many will display greater potential for comorbid symptoms of oppositional defiant disorder, conduct disorder, depression, and anxiety (Biederman & Steingard, 1989; Faigel et al., 1995; Robin, 1998; Wender, 1995). Certainly, adolescents in therapy demonstrate more developed verbal and interactive skills than younger children or preadolescents. However, the benefits gained by engaging these skills are often offset by the intensity and severity of behavioral symptoms associated with both the ADHD and other comorbid disorders (see Table 7.1).

THE RANGE OF CLINICAL INTERVENTIONS
FOR ADOLESCENTS WITH ADHD

Clinical interventions for ADHD adolescents follow the general range of interventions that we described for ADHD children in Chapter 6. However, with adolescents, we focus more on family interactions, parent and sibling issues, the adolescent's social and academic struggles, and self-esteem building. The frequency and timing of these interventions is also different. We continue to place great importance on the involvement of and consultation with parents; indeed, when treating adolescents, we conduct more joint sessions with the adolescent present than we would with ADHD children. These joint sessions involve discussion of the adolescent's and the family's history, test results, medication issues, and treatment planning. The therapist must work to

TABLE 7.1. Differential Clinical Features of ADHD Adolescents Compared to ADHD Children

1. Greater accumulated personal discouragement and frustration.
2. Greater awareness of their personal difficulties.
3. Greater awareness of their "differentness" from siblings and peers.
4. Less self-confidence and lower self-esteem.
5. Greater confusion in response to educational experiences beginning in middle school.
6. Greater degrees of distractibility apparent from the beginning of middle school.
7. Greater educational challenges and frustrations.
8. Greater risk for school failure or dropping out.
9. Greater risk of legal implications for hyperactive–impulsive behaviors.
10. Greater experiences of accumulated parental frustration.
11. Greater risk of potential parental and/or family violence.
12. Higher risk for comorbid symptoms of oppositional defiant disorder, conduct disorder, depression, and anxiety.

make the young adolescent feel valued and respected as a contributor in these areas of information gathering and decision making. The therapist must help the adolescent build self-esteem and facilitate her or his process of maturation. We have found that the more an ADHD adolescent feels included in the early therapy process, the better the outcome for that adolescent. During joint sessions, the interchanges that occur between parents and their adolescents can foster a new rapport and mutual respect.

We also devote more time to individual sessions with ADHD adolescents because of the need to grapple with issues of independence and self-discipline in a context that builds self-esteem. As noted, many ADHD adolescents continue to be quite immature (compared to their non-ADHD peers), even up to age 16. We have found that carefully designed individual and even family-oriented "play" activities can be quite effective in engaging such immature adolescents. Enlisting the ADHD adolescent's high energy in a competitive or interactive experience (e.g., shooting baskets, throwing darts, or playing a game) provides the adolescent with new opportunities for success. (These "active" sessions are more useful for the hyperactive–impulsive ADHD type adolescents than for the more inattentive-type individuals, who tend to be less active and competitive.) We often balance individual play-activity sessions with one-on-one conversations in our office.

Work with ADHD adolescents also involves their role within their family system. After some progress has been made individually with the adolescent and concurrently with their parents, we conduct family therapy sessions. Unlike our procedure with ADHD children, we often conduct a sibling session, that is, a session with the siblings and the ADHD adolescent together, without their parents. This kind of session gives the therapist an overview of sibling interaction patterns, the extent of scapegoating, the maturity levels of the other siblings, their definition of their own roles in the family, and their perceptions of their parents. Therapist observations regarding these issues are important for setting goals and developing interventions for the whole family. This early sibling session also fosters the development of sibling comfort and identification with the therapist before the family sessions begin. These family sessions continue until the ADHD adolescent's role in the family is normalized to some extent and the parents feel more in control of the family. Given success in these family sessions, marital therapy and intergenerational sessions are conducted, if necessary. These essentially follow the same format described for ADHD children in Chapter 6. The clinical sequence that we will discuss is outlined in Table 7.2.

TABLE 7.2. A Clinical Sequence for the Evaluation and Treatment of ADHD Adolescents and Their Families

Session	Format
1	Parents only
2–3	Adolescent individually
4	Feedback with parents only
5–6	Family: parent–adolescent
7–10	Adolescent individually
10+	Siblings
	Nuclear family
	Intergenerational system
	Marriage

A TREATMENT MODEL FOR ADOLESCENTS WITH ADHD AND THEIR FAMILIES

Session 1: Parents Only

The initial session is focused on goals similar to the ones we discussed in working with ADHD children in Chapter 6. The initial interview with parents by themselves is critical in establishing a level of rapport that cannot be achieved as easily with the ADHD adolescent present. Parents need an opportunity to vent their frustrations and fears. Most parents will be more candid and open without the adolescent present. However, some parents misuse the initial therapy session to scapegoat their child, telling the therapist how "bad" their youngster has become. This separate interview with the parents also protects the adolescent from these dynamics being repeated in the therapy session.

Of course, there are exceptions to holding the initial interview with the parent alone. In an immediate crisis involving suicidal ideation or suicide attempts, or if the adolescent is out of control physically, several initial sessions with the adolescent individually, or with the adolescent and the parents jointly, might be necessary to stabilize the adolescent before ongoing therapy commences.

The overall goal of this initial session with the parents is to explore the developmental history of the adolescent as a child, including his or her medical, social, and educational experiences from infancy to the present, as discussed in Chapter 6. A review of the family's history and development should follow the outline presented earlier in Table 6.2. In this initial parent session the therapist must respond genuinely to the parents' concerns and struggles and begin establishing a cooperative relationship that conveys optimism and hope.

Sessions 2 and 3: The Adolescent Individually

These next two individual sessions with the adolescent are intended to establish a relationship with the adolescent and to gain a firsthand understanding of the range and expression of the ADHD symptoms. The therapist explores the youngster's perceptions of her or his roles at home, in school, and socially with peers. With younger or more immature adolescents, the initial session usually begins in the office setting but may conclude with the last 15 to 20 minutes in what we call our "active playroom." We often move from the office to this playroom as a means of surprising the adolescent with a different and more engaging setting that generates a greater level of ease. This sequence also establishes early expectations in the adolescent that talking about issues occurs in the office before moving to the playroom, where the adolescent can then relate to the therapist in a different context.

We described the makeup of our playroom for young children in Chapter 6. This room is equipped with a number of board and card games, bean bags, stuffed animals, a Nerf basketball hoop, several safe dart games on the walls, and a 5-foot-tall canvas punching/kicking bag. Play can be very effective for the more active and restless ADHD adolescent who has difficulty sitting still in the therapist's office and engaging in one-on-one conversation for an hour. This open-ended yet controlled setting not only gives the youngster something active to do that is challenging, but it also provides a comfortable form of interaction—and occasionally competition—with the therapist. Since many hyperactive–impulsive adolescents tend to be competitive, their efforts to beat the therapist in a game of shooting baskets or throwing darts can be quite engaging.

For many ADHD adolescents, this playroom experience can elicit, in a single session, a meaningful dimension of trust and rapport with the therapist that might have taken 6 to 8 weeks to build via one-on-one conversations in the office. In this kind of setting with ADHD adolescents the therapist's skills as a play therapist do not need to be as refined (in terms of understanding symbolic play and expression) as they should be when working with ADHD children, especially very young ones. The focus of this play experience is to provide the ADHD adolescent with an acceptable means of actively expressing behaviors that can occur with the therapist. This experience coaxes trust and interaction from even the most resistant adolescents. Many youngsters who would otherwise sit mutely in an office—fidgeting, playing with the chair, twisting their clothes, or looking out the window—will talk nonstop about both mundane and serious issues in their lives while they are shooting baskets or throwing darts.

This form of play therapy is quite distinct from the more tradi-tional approaches in which the play is the vehicle for the therapy and its symbolic messages are the therapist's focus. Our use of active play with ADHD adolescents provides a structured context for essentially cognitive interactions—we often refer to this process as "therapy while playing." The play activities have the effect of focusing and channeling the adolescent's energy while dissipating layers of anxiety that can impede the progress of effective verbal exchanges in the more formal office setting. In other words, this method creates a more appealing context for personal interaction and the exploration of cognitive issues as the therapeutic relationship unfolds.

Inevitably, the therapist will be drawn into the competitive games available in the playroom. Managed properly, this experience can help build identification and trust. Many parents of 14- and 15-year-old children tell us that their youngsters look forward to coming to the therapy appointments because they enjoy playing darts or basketball with the therapist. Some of the more aggressive and frustrated adoles-cents (females as well as males) will put on the boxing gloves and hit and kick the large punching bag mercilessly while the therapist holds it steady for them. We invite the parents of some of these students to come in to observe the aggression that their child is taking out on the punching bag; sometimes we suggest that the parents consider buying a small punching bag to hang at home.

The value of focusing the ADHD adolescent's restlessness and aggression on the punching bag instead of objects at home or even sib-lings is obvious. We do not agree with the opinion, often voiced by parents, teachers, and other therapists, that this type of activity may "reinforce aggression." It has been our consistent experience that refo-cusing the adolescent's energy and aggression in a manner more acceptable to parents and teachers enhances both self-control and self-esteem.

Many parents of ADHD adolescents, particularly those who dis-play more inattentive than hyperactive symptoms, are often amazed at the energy and aggression that their child can display. One mother, who was in the playroom watching her daughter hit and kick the punching bag, said to the therapist, "I can't watch this anymore. It scares me. I've never seen her like this," and then left the playroom. The therapist spent the last 10 minutes of the session with the mother, helping her to digest her own responses to this aggressive side of her primarily inattentive daughter. She had never witnessed her daughter in a rage, though she had received reports from school about her occa-sional eruptions that often led to fights with her peers. The whole punching bag experience also reminded the mother of her older brother who, during their years growing up together, would often verbally and physically threaten her and her parents. Some weeks later she and the therapist concluded that her brother probably had undiagnosed ADHD. This link to her own distressing experiences opened the door for the mother to understand her daughter's struggles. Thereafter she tried to find ways of relating to her daughter that would help her daughter to express her frustrations and dissatisfactions openly rather than bury them inside her. The mother also realized that she had been attempting to protect her ADHD daughter—and also herself—from these aggressive behaviors.

In Chapter 2 we discussed research indicating that adolescent ADHD males display considerably more impulsive–hyperactive symptoms than their female counterparts, and that ADHD females display more inattentive characteristics than males. While some of these girls may evidence fidgety and restless behaviors, they usually do not have the same intense need for physical activity as the ADHD boys do. In fact, many of these young girls can be quite passive, displaying more depressive symptoms. These girls may be described by their teachers and school counselors as "flaky," "scatterbrained," or "spacey." These characterizations reflect adults' frustrations with these adolescents' difficulties in paying attention in the classroom or staying "on track" in their conversations. Most of these inattentive-type adolescents are usually more responsive to clinical work and interaction in the office setting, one-on-one, than the hyperactive–impulsive adolescents.

A high school junior was referred for depression by his pediatrician, who had diagnosed and medicated him several years earlier with ADHD, inattentive type. He sullenly stared at the floor throughout his first session with the therapist. Consequently, the therapist decided to hold the second session in the playroom. To the therapist's surprise, the new patient, unlike most ADHD adolescent boys, was not interested in engaging in any of the available activities. The therapist learned that the boy had never been successful athletically and tended to avoid any type of competition. Even tossing a ball seemed intimidating to him.

The therapist sat on a beanbag chair in the playroom as the junior reluctantly discussed his lack of friends and sense of loneliness. He was an only child living with his single mother, whose work caused her to travel several days a week. His father had left when he was young, and his grandfather, to whom he had become quite bonded, had died a year earlier. At one point he mentioned that he and his grandfather had played checkers a lot and that his grandfather had been teaching him to play chess just before he died. The therapist promptly got out a checker board, and they played together for the remainder of the session. By the third session the patient had become more comfortable and confident playing checkers. This was an acceptable diversion that allowed him to be more open, and at times, even humorous. In the beginning of their play, he never looked up at the therapist but focused only on the checkers. However, he managed to share much about himself and his family experiences while intently studying the checker board.

By the fourth session he asked if they could meet in the therapist's office with the checker board because the playroom was too distracting for him. Thereafter, he would arrive for his individual appointment, eager and often smiling, with this immediate request: "Can we play checkers today?" As they talked, the therapist learned more about the student's struggles and discouragement in school and developed a plan with the youngster to request some specific accommodations in his classrooms. In addition, the student revealed that he did not think that the Ritalin he was taking doing any good, though he remembered that it had helped him "focus" several years ago when it was first prescribed. The therapist called the boy's physician, the medication was changed to Dexedrine, and the change produced remarkably positive results. Within several weeks the patient was able to boast of improved grades and more confidence in school. He even joined a community soccer league, which was less competitive than the school's varsity team. Gradually, he learned that he could keep up physically and compete with his peers. In fact, his mother expressed surprise at his level of aggression on the soccer field. In addition to dealing with the ADHD symptoms, this student needed more individual help to process his grief over the loss of his father and grandfather. Much of his natural aggressiveness seemed to have been tucked away (repressed) with the grief and underlying anger associated with the early loss of his father.

Session 4: Parents' Feedback

This session is typically conducted without the ADHD adolescent present. The goal is to help the parents understand and assimilate the implications of their child's symptoms, whether or not the ADHD diagnosis has been made by this time. The therapist provides the parents with observations of the clinical interviews and impressions regarding the range of the adolescent's symptoms. This may involve introducing explicit issues related to the ADHD disorder as well as identifying potential comorbid symptoms. This feedback session can be a pivotal session in that it allows parents to work through their anger and frustration regarding their adolescent's long-term struggles, failures, and disruptive behaviors. The parents often need the privacy of this separate session to talk freely about, and deal with, their accumulated feelings. If ADHD is unfamiliar to the parents, the therapist will need to provide basic information and details about the disorder. It is always important to identify explicitly for the parents the effects that these symptoms have had on their adolescent's development and the family's interactions.

This session also focuses on parental roles and strategies. In addition to introducing the parent management issues discussed in Chapter 6, the therapist must identify normal adolescent behaviors and distinguish them from ADHD symptoms. We find it helpful to elicit the parents' experiences when they were adolescents. The symptoms identified in Table 7.1 are discussed in the context of the parents' growing frustrations with their child. More realistic goals for parenting are explored in an effort to increase objectivity and reduce their discouragement. Their youngster's behaviors are also discussed more objectively in the context of her or his role in the family and with siblings. This session prepares the parents to handle the ensuing sessions with their ADHD adolescent present. It also serves to strengthen the alliance between the parents and the therapist. This is important to the following family therapy sessions for a variety of reasons: (1) it gives the parents hope, (2) it confirms their feelings and frustrations, (3) it gives them a feeling of working jointly with a professional, and (4) it provides the therapist with resources to intervene more effectively (blocking negativity and scapegoating, when necessary, or providing support when they consider giving up).

Sessions 5 and 6: The Initial Family Sessions

These two sessions, conducted jointly with the ADHD adolescent and the parents, (but without the siblings), are focused on defining and clearly elucidating the impact of ADHD on the adolescent and within the family's daily (and past) life experiences. There are several goals here:

1. Review the ADHD diagnosis and its ramifications on the adolescent and elicit parental support.
2. Review psychoeducational testing data.
3. Block and extinguish any continuing parental scapegoating of the ADHD adolescent.
4. Reduce distancing behaviors between parents and adolescent.
5. Develop a parent–adolescent behavioral expectation plan and continuing treatment plan.

Goal 1

With the information and support of the prior session "under their belts," the parents should now be able to offer more understanding and empathy to their adolescent regarding her or his symptoms and struggles. Even parents who are still highly frustrated by and discouraged with their child's problems can become somewhat supportive once they understand that there is a biological cause for their child's problematic behaviors. Parents can also look back over their adolescent's early development and grade school years with increased understanding. Often a poignant empathy for what their child has endured becomes apparent.

The identification of the diagnosis can also be used therapeutically with the adolescent. In this session we focus on the biochemical and medical aspects of ADHD. This serves as a reminder to parents and gives the adolescent a new way of understanding her or his prior struggles and behaviors. Some therapists, and parents, might worry that this approach be put to negative use by youngsters as an "excuse" or justification for their problem behaviors. However, we find that most adolescents are relieved to know that there is a biological reason for their struggles and that they are not "stupid," or "bad," or "crazy." This is the beginning, therapeutically, of rebuilding parental ties and self-esteem for the adolescent. (In Session 10, to follow, we will describe how the diagnosis is used therapeutically to challenge scapegoating in families.)

Adolescents may resist the diagnosis of ADHD for a variety of reasons. Some are afraid of being stigmatized, of being viewed as even more different at a time in their lives when they are trying to fit in and be accepted by their peers. Others fear that they will be labeled "dumb" or be put in "special" classes. Still others worry that if they take medications, everyone in the school will find out and ridicule them because of it. Many of these adolescents already know that other students go to the school nurse's office regularly to take their medications. (The sustained-release stimulant medications are often preferred for ADHD adolescents because they eliminate the need for a midday dosage.)

These parent–adolescent sessions provide an opportunity for the airing of concerns and fears by both the parents and the adolescent. The therapist can address these concerns and allay fears by providing honest, clear answers. Moreover, the therapist has the opportunity to encourage and, if necessary, move the parents into more supportive roles, that may be very new to them. As discussed in Chapter 6, catalyzing the parents' willingness to participate in a supportive and understanding manner can be a powerful intervention. Many ADHD adolescents express relief in these sessions when their parents finally "see" their pain and struggles. For many families these joint sessions open the door to healing and further constructive therapeutic work together.

Goal 2

If the testing has been completed by the time these sessions are held, it should be reviewed. We have found that it is therapeutically essential to review test results simultaneously with the ADHD adolescent and her or his parents. The therapist needs to ensure that the *same information* is shared with everyone to preclude future misunderstandings or misinterpretations. It also provides an opportunity for the adolescent and the parents to look at the data together, ask questions, and begin to process the fact that the youngster has clear strengths in some areas and deficits in others. It is important for the therapist who is not experienced in working with testing data to carefully review of the results in the context of *both* apparent strengths and deficits. Now is the time to say something like, "Even though there are some low scores in these areas, you should be pleased that your performance scores on the IQ test are so high" or, "Look at the high percentile scores that you achieved in expressive language compared to these scores in short-term memory."

The test data need to be translated for the adolescent and parents into comprehensible language. Implications regarding school functioning and future achievement should be discussed. This leads naturally to consideration of the need for classroom accommodations. We have developed several lists of possible academic accommodations (see Appendices 3.2 and 3.3 in Chapter 3, pages 93 and 94, respectively) for the educational settings of middle and high school ADHD students. At this point in the session, we often give one of these lists to the youngster and her or his parents. Most parents have little awareness of why accommodations would be requested, what the goals are, or what practical accommodations really involve. This discussion of accommodations can be continued at a later date, for example, when a teacher conference or a "504" meeting is scheduled. Prior to a school conference, the therapist would meet individually with the adolescent to review specific classroom and study experiences, and prepare a list of relevant accommodations to be recommended.

Goal 3

It is important to identify and block the embedded patterns of scapegoating that may continue to be directed at the ADHD adolescent even in the face of understanding of the diagnosis by the parents. As the therapist objectifies this dynamic by interrupting the parents' critical or blaming remarks, the adolescent experiences a new sense of relief. When the parents begin to see the hurtful reality underlying their scapegoating behavior, they not only gain more control over it but also recognize such behavior when it comes from the non-ADHD siblings. The therapist must make progress in blocking this scapegoating in these early sessions with the parents, before the sibling(s) are included, so that the parents can be more supportive of the ADHD youngster and less reinforcing of those dynamics with the other children.

Goal 4

The long-term conflict and discouragement experienced by the parents of an ADHD adolescent creates substantial distancing in addition to the scapegoating. This distancing can be observed in both the emotional and the physical arenas. Of course, this distancing is usually reciprocated by the ADHD adolescent, who has learned to use distance as a protective mechanism. When the parents and the adolescent arrive for sessions in the therapist's office, it is not unusual to find them choosing seats at some distance from one another. The therapist must begin the process of reducing barriers and provide opportunities for mutual positive engagement.

We described the use of the active playroom previously. Occasionally we will use this setting with the adolescent and her or his parents to aid the engagement experience. For example, this setting enables angry and withdrawn parents (particularly the attacking parent) to interact with their youngster in a supervised and safe environment. Play can be more powerful than talk. Often the therapist encourages the parent to try shooting some baskets or throwing some darts with her or his adolescent. These activities are pursued with a parent only after the adolescent has accrued individual experience in the playroom, has learned the therapist's rules and limits, and has gained some self-control and constraint in the activities. Usually these adolescents are quick to engage their parents in the activity that they *know* they can win. We have found that, in this particular context, it is better to involve only one parent at a time. Typically, we choose the more distant, authoritarian, or attacking parent because he or she habitually avoids playful interaction with his or her child. However, sometimes we also involve the protective parent if she or he has never engaged the adolescent in any direct (and safe) competition. The therapist becomes the observer, scorekeeper, and monitor of the level of intensity, intervening when the adolescent becomes too aggressive or "wild" with the parent.

Playroom activity shared by parents and adolescent is dramatically more effective when only one parent is present at a time; this configuration bypasses broader parental and family roles and supports a one-on-one experience. When both parents are present in the play-room, the adolescent tends to focus on getting attention from the more distant parent, occasionally playing the parents against one another, and often replicating the everyday conflicts of this parent–child sub-system. Some adolescents may also feel overwhelmed by being the only child in a room with three adults.

The use of this active play environment with both parents can also trigger underlying rivalries between the parents themselves. The respective protector and disciplinarian roles, or other underlying mari-tal conflicts, can spill over into the activities with the adolescent. In other words, many parents of ADHD adolescents simply cannot play well together.

Goal 5

Toward the end of these sessions, it is important for the therapist to help the parents and the ADHD adolescent negotiate a mutual plan concerning everyday behaviors and expectations at home. For exam-ple, the discussion regarding this plan may involve a redefinition of the adolescent's household chores so that they are clear to him or her. We often suggest that they be out in writing and posted in a special location, and that they be defined by a time table. Rewards, such as an allowance, television and computer time, and telephone access are also outlined. A clear curfew is established, and expectations regarding the youngster's interactions with the parents and siblings are discussed. The goal is for the parents and the adolescent to discuss these matters objectively and straightforwardly, and then to create a realistic and acceptable plan together. Their past attempts to discuss such issues may have ended in punitive threats by a parent and angry remarks by the adolescent. The goal of this plan is to foster both a sense of control for the parents and to identify a range of expectations for the adoles-cent. A good plan should reduce stress and chaos in the family while furthering therapeutic changes.

Finally, the ongoing treatment plan is reviewed with the adoles-cent. Since most of the assessment has been completed by this stage, it is time to move on to a combination of individual sessions with the adolescent and family sessions with the parents and siblings present.

Sessions 7–10: The Adolescent Individually

If the prior sessions with the parents alone and with the parents and ADHD adolescent have been successful, the family environment gas been stabilized. The parents are now considerably more understanding of the disorder and its impact on the affected child, the siblings, the family as a whole, and their marital relationship. However, these initial sessions may have also identified other concerns for the parents, such as the pressing need to refocus on their other children's activities and behaviors and on their own marriage. This refocusing shifts excessive parental attention away from the ADHD adolescent and reduces reactive emotions within the family. If the parents are still having difficulty with issues related to the ADHD or continuing conflict with the adolescent's behaviors, concurrent sessions may be scheduled to address these issues.

Most ADHD adolescents recognize and appreciate that their parents have settled down. They are pleased that they are no longer subject to negative scrutiny. Their sense of relief frees them to deal with their school struggles, both educationally and socially. With parents who continue to be overly intrusive, the therapist must be persistent in insisting that they back off, particularly from overscrutinizing or continuing to scapegoat their adolescent. Enforcing boundaries for both parents and adolescent allows the therapist to deal with the adolescent more effectively and on a more personal level for several weeks. Of course, the long-term goal is to develop new roles and skills with the parents so that they become more effective in helping and supporting their adolescent.

These individual sessions with the adolescent focus initially on practical aspects of modifying school pressures and behavior problems. The therapist discusses concrete ways to organize time and materials, prepare assignments, and study for tests. This leads to discussions of how to structure and manage time at home, which in turn might surface more painful issues of how the adolescent relates to his or her parents and siblings. Often the ADHD adolescent expresses considerable anger at, and disappointment about, these chronically difficult family relationships. Social relationships and dating are also discussed, particularly in terms of how ADHD symptoms may affect the adolescent's experiences. The goal, of course, is to help the adolescent create successful experiences that foster an optimistic sense of the future.

A 16-year-old adolescent was brought to the therapist (SVE) by her exasperated parents who were concerned because she was unhappy and depressed. The girl's behavior and moods had changed dramatically over the past year. Although she had never been much invested in school, she had previously appeared to care about her grades and to make an effort to complete her work. However, her parents acknowledged that even in grade school she had seemed "unfocused" and had taken longer to complete homework than seemed necessary. This year she had begun to skip school and did not even attempt to complete her homework. She had recently begun to wear black clothes and nail polish, and had colored her blond hair black. The parents reported that she seemed interested in the occult and was often preoccupied by issues of death and the afterlife. Many of her friends used drugs, and she had admitted to her parents that she was experimenting with marijuana. At home she isolated herself in her room and was distant and unresponsive. She was now failing several of her classes but did not appear to care.

In the therapist's office the girl sat with a dreamy expression on her face, appearing calm and serene. She was an attractive young lady but did not seem to recognize this herself. She spoke of herself in disparaging ways, saying that she was a failure and utterly unable to please her parents or herself. She believed that she was "stupid" and acknowledged having given up on schoolwork because nothing she did was successful or gained her good grades. She talked positively only about a few friends. She could not think about a future, let alone ponder goals or ambitions. When she was asked about suicidal thoughts, she admitted that there had been times when she had considered "ending it." She showed the therapist some of her poetry, which was filled with dark thoughts and tortured imagery.

It would have been reasonable clinically to focus solely on the girl's depressive, even morbid, demeanor. However, her early school history and level of academic frustrations suggested other possibilities. The overlay of depression masked underlying ADHD symptoms. The results of private testing indicated a clear pattern of ADHD in an extremely bright adolescent. Neither she nor her parents were able to accept the positive elements of her intellectual resources from the test data at this point. The psychiatrist prescribed a stimulant medication. He wanted to see what effect the stimulant medication might have before considering the addition of an antidepressant medication.

Within a couple of weeks the changes in her behavior were quite dramatic. She reported feeling more focused and settled at school and at home. Gradually she began to wear more varied and colorful clothing and even gave up her black nail polish and hair dye. She was surprised that she could remember more things at school, and her homework seemed to come more easily for her. Her grades rapidly began to improve, and she began to interact with her parents and siblings in a more cordial manner. Her parents were grateful that they "had gotten their daughter back." She reported that she had lost many of her old friends when she stopped dressing in black and skipping her classes, but she also noted that she was making some new friends. Therapy moved from several parent–adolescent sessions to three family sessions with her and the other siblings. These helped clarify changes she had made and repair negative images and behaviors with her two younger siblings. Two individual sessions with the adolescent were interspersed to assist her with self-esteem and self-confidence issues. The therapy process terminated in about 4 months.

Clearly the depression was secondary to the underlying and long-term ADHD, and no antidepressant medications were necessary. By the end of therapy she was talking with her parents for the first time about attending college.

As we have noted, many ADHD adolescents have difficulty considering future goals and choices. Most seem afraid to consider college or even life after high school. We have found that it is important to discuss future training and education with them. Often the therapist will be the first adult to ask them—without nagging, warning, or criticizing—about their thoughts regarding college or careers. Usually these youngsters are willing to share their doubts and fears about the future with the therapist because they perceive the therapist as less judgmental than their parents.

If the ADHD adolescent requires help and advocacy in the school setting, the therapist should spend one of these individual sessions reviewing our model accommodations lists and writing a similar list that precisely identifies the areas of difficulty for this particular student. This list may note specific needs, for example, with certain teachers and in certain classrooms, and general needs, for example, systemwide adjustments for all reading assignments or for all test situations. It has been our experience that when the parents, student, and therapist arrive for a "504" or IEP conference at the school with no such clear and detailed plan in hand, too much time is spent reviewing the student's behaviors and puzzling over the teachers' observations and struggles, leaving inadequate time at the end of the meeting to produce educational plans and accommodations that have specificity and relevance for the ADHD student.

We believe that it is more effective to develop this list without the parents present because the adolescent will be more candid about her or his actual school experiences. The therapist should encourage the adolescent to honestly describe the types of frustrations and struggles he or she encounters, so that true barriers to learning can be identified and realistic accommodations requested. The adolescent and therapist reach a consensus regarding what will be communicated to the schools regarding the student's problems and academic needs. This session also prepares the student to articulate her or his struggles with teachers in the meeting. (Some schools will routinely exclude a student from these meetings. We always stipulate that the student should be present to explain their own experiences and engage in dialogue with the teachers.)

Several days prior to the meeting this "proposed accommodations list" is faxed to the appropriate individual at the school (e.g., the school psychologist or counselor) and it is also mailed to the parents. The list communicates to school personnel the seriousness of the therapist and parents regarding the upcoming conference and provides an immediate source of structure for the meeting. Most school personnel are happy to have such input to help prepare a written educational plan. Occasionally, however, the therapist will encounter a school psychologist or special education director who is offended by the suggested accommodations list, usually because she or he perceives it as an intrusion into her or his areas of expertise. This is why we try to keep the presentation of the list somewhat casual and why we deliberately identify it as a "proposed list." However, it is important for the therapist, as an advocate, to remain firm even when dealing with an offended school staff person. In 90% of these situations, the school personnel thank us for providing consultation and specific recommendations and compliment the ADHD student for being so well prepared and reflective in the meeting.

These individual sessions may need to be continued for some time for adolescents with comorbid symptoms of oppositional defiant disorder, conduct disorder, depression, or anxiety in order to address these difficulties. For example, the 16-year-old girl described in the case example was seen in several additional individual sessions, even after the medication assisted her in school, so that the therapist could monitor and help her understand her depressive symptoms and suicidal thoughts. The therapist worked to teach her how to recognize these comorbid symptoms quickly, should they recur. When additional focused individual sessions are deemed necessary, they may be interspersed with the family sessions.

Sessions 10+: Family Therapy Sessions

Sibling Subsystem

After some of the above goals have been met, particularly the goals of promoting family stabilization and cooperation between parents and the ADHD adolescent, a meeting with the siblings and the ADHD adolescent (A sibling interaction session) can be productive. Some experienced family therapists may feel that such a meeting should come earlier, closer to the beginning of the treatment process. We agree with that reasoning for other general clinical situations. However, we have found that, regarding ADHD, if a sibling session is held prematurely, before early stabilization and improvement of family interaction has occurred, one of two undesirable outcomes is likely: angry, frustrated siblings will spend the entire session scapegoating the ADHD adolescent or they will remain silent and withholding out of fear of becoming too angry, losing control, and saying the "wrong things." Similarly, we have also learned that it is often not effective, or even safe, to engage the ADHD adolescent in playroom activities with adolescent-age siblings. The underlying sibling rivalries and jealousies can easily erupt and quickly escalate to chaotic, if not destructive, proportions. In such a volatile situation the therapist too often gets pulled into a controlling and often scolding parental role that is countertherapeutic.

When the scapegoating dynamic has been embedded in the roles and image system of the family system for a decade or more, reactivity toward the ADHD youngster may still be present even after initial improvements in the family have occurred. Delaying the sibling interaction session until these positive changes are more firmly anchored gives the therapist more leverage to challenge the siblings' habituated responses toward their ADHD sister or brother. Having gained some relief from patterns they thought would never change, siblings should be more willing to look at the broader family functioning with some objectivity and should be eager to begin to repair their relationships with their ADHD sibling. If this first sibling session is a constructive session, several more may be scheduled consecutively, as needed.

Time spent with the siblings aids the therapist in understanding their attitudes and behaviors with one another (free of the presence of their parents), fosters a sense of rapport that can be important in the family sessions, and helps the therapist intervene more effectively if the family's long-term pattern of scapegoating emerges in the ensuing family sessions.

Nuclear Family Sessions

These sessions involving everyone in the nuclear family—the parents, the siblings, and the ADHD adolescent—are important for redefining the perceptions and functioning of the family as a system. Often the therapist must create new structural patterns for the family and help all the family members delineate new boundaries. In some cases the pattern of parental intrusiveness and/or parental–sibling scapegoating of the ADHD adolescent is deeply entrenched. If the family dynamics feel too chaotic to the therapist, he or she should schedule an additional session with the parents by themselves to help them gain a better sense of parental adequacy, as well as one or two additional sibling sessions to give these youngsters more time to vent their continuing grievances and learn how to manage them. As the parents' attitudes about themselves and their role in the family improves, the imbedded scapegoating and criticism of the ADHD adolescent will subside.

These family sessions begin by reviewing what has been learned about ADHD symptoms and their impact on the family's relationships and overall functioning. As the family is assembling in the office, the therapist invites the ADHD adolescent to take the chair next to the therapist. This seating strategy immediately announces to the family that the ADHD adolescent is receiving support from the therapist. At one level, this alignment sends a message to the parents and siblings that the therapist will intervene to block scapegoating if it occurs. At another level, the alignment suggests that the family can move beyond the scapegoating and recognize the new status accorded to the ADHD adolescent by the therapist. In addition, the ADHD adolescent's proximity allows the therapist to manage his or her reactive or defensive responses to the family's interaction more directly, to offer more immediate support, and occasionally to refocus the adolescent's attention, for example, by touching her or his chair or making eye contact. This intervention is usually only necessary in the first family session.

In the subsequent family sessions the therapist's goal is to steer the exchanges away from ADHD issues, since they should have been discussed thoroughly in the initial family interview, and redirect the focus toward the everyday patterns of interaction and communication in the family. This therapeutic intervention is intended to divert too exclusive attention on the ADHD adolescent and normalize her or his role in the family's daily life experiences. These sessions can also provide the parents with an opportunity to practice their improved coparenting roles with the entire family present. Parent–child issues, such as dealing with siblings' needs for attention or privacy or for increased time with one or both parents, can be similarly addressed.

In some families where the dysfunctional patterns (particularly the scapegoating) are rigidly embedded, more focused interventions aimed at diffusing the ADHD symptoms are necessary. Unlike family therapy that focuses primarily on behavioral or interactive problems, the therapist working with an ADHD family can point to a rather specific biological etiology. At one level, this use of the diagnosis may seem to reinforce the family's scapegoating behaviors by "agreeing" that there is "something wrong" with the ADHD child. However, at another level it diffuses the scapegoating by providing a medical explanation for the problem behaviors rather than for the variety of reasons that can be cited as causes of the scapegoating process (personality flaws, differentness, craziness, or parental failure). The therapeutic issue in these family therapy sessions is different from that in the initial session with the parents, when the therapist was responsible for explaining the diagnosis based on accurate theory and research. Here the therapist moves to a more strategic therapeutic role by dramatizing the diagnosis in a manner that removes or diffuses the negative perceptions attached to the ADHD child. This goal can be accomplished over the course of several therapeutic interventions:

1. Explain the diagnosis in a context of other medical conditions that elicits more concern, and even sympathy, from family members toward the ADHD adolescent. We use analogous conditions such as diabetes or other chronic disabilities. For example, we may recount a case involving a diabetic adolescent who must take insulin each day to survive. Often, family members readily identify with the sufferer and her or his family's response to that member. For most families this challenges their perceptions of the ADHD family member and quickly diffuses the scapegoating by providing opportunities for more empathic relating.

2. With families who display more rigid scapegoating or chaotic interactions, the diagnosis needs to be dramatized such that it is "bigger than life." We may introduce more technical issues regarding neurology and brain chemistry and provide copies of research articles (recognizing that most family members will not understand or care about these details). In very difficult families we may hypothetically "create" and attach a medical condition to a parent or sibling as another way of deflecting the attention on the scapegoated child. For example, we may say, "What do you all think would happen to your family if your dad were injured in an automobile accident and could no longer work or even care for himself ?" Or, "What would it be like if your sister were injured and her leg had to be amputated ?" The goal is twofold: (a) to make the diagnosis so dramatic that it can no longer be used against the adolescent, and (b) to deflect the family's attention, at least temporarily, from scapegoating the ADHD member.

3. With other families it can be helpful to discuss the family's leisure activities—or, more often, the total lack of such activities. Typically, focusing on this topic initially elicits underlying feelings of neglect and a quick tendency to blame the ADHD sibling for the absence of family time together. The therapist can help the dysfunctional family plan a trip together or even subgroup activities, for example, the father could take the older children fishing, while the mother took the younger children to the park. This kind of planning can "normalize" the family, communicating that it is healthy enough to do more normal activities together with their ADHD member. Of course, this kind of planning also communicates to the ADHD adolescent a new sense of acceptance in the family. These family sessions establish

new pathways of relating that improve overall family functioning as well as repairing the long-term conflicts and wounds between members.

Intergenerational Family Sessions

These sessions, most often involving grandparents, are used less frequently with ADHD adolescents than with ADHD children simply because grandparents are typically less involved with their adolescent grandchildren. Of course, there are exceptions that would necessitate their involvement: for example, grandparents (or other extended family members) who live in the family's household or highly involved or intrusive grandparents who participate in the family's everyday life. Grandparents who have made a considerable emotional, and often financial, investment in their grandchildren "being successful," attending a specific college, or pursuing a certain career, may need to be included if they exert significant influence on the family dynamics— whether they live nearby or out of state.

Family therapists may be familiar with more typical "family-of-origin consultations," particularly those used in marital therapy to gain information and feedback about the spouses' early roles and growing-up experiences (see Framo, 1992). The goals of these family-of-origin sessions for ADHD adolescents are more educationally oriented. The therapist's role is to inform the grandparents of the meaning of the diagnosis and the ongoing treatment plan and to articulate the adolescent's needs in the family. The therapist may address the supportive roles grandparents can perform with the adolescent or, conversely, the therapist may need to help the parents set boundaries to limit the grandparents' criticism and/or intrusiveness into the nuclear family.

In the context of working with ADHD families, the involvement of the grandparents, or other significantly involved extended family members, is both psychoeducational and interventional. The grandparents need to have the same information about ADHD, its origins and effects, as do the adolescent, the parents, and the siblings. The disorder should be framed in a realistic context that also conveys a hopeful treatment outcome. Many grandparents mistakenly blame their adult children's "poor parenting" for their grandchild's behavioral and academic problems. Others participate in the scapegoating dynamics of the nuclear family. In such cases the therapist might have to schedule several sessions with the parents, the ADHD adolescent, and the grandparents to provide interventions that diffuse the patterns of blaming and/or scapegoating in which the grandparents have participated. Often, once the grandparents recognize that the parents have begun to understand and relate to the ADHD adolescent in a different manner and that the adolescent is functioning within the family more appropriately, they alter their own attitudes and behaviors.

Marital Therapy

Sessions focused on the spouses' relationship can become an important resource for the parents of ADHD adolescents. Unfortunately, many therapists and school counselors who provide evaluations of ADHD children and adolescents rarely address or have the training to offer aid or referrals to the parents for marital assistance. Their clinical focus is directed solely at the ADHD child or adolescent, exclusive of the broader family struggles. *We strongly believe that if the above therapeutic interventions with ADHD families are to be effective and lasting, marital therapy must be provided for the parents.* In Chapters 4 and 5 we outlined how the patterns of accumulating stress in parents of ADHD children gradually spill over into their marital interactions, eroding their bonding and intimacy. Typically, by the time an ADHD child has reached adolescence, 8 to 10 years of parent–child difficulties have strained spouses' personal connection to one another to the breaking point.

Once the ADHD child enters puberty, parents are faced with a new layer of typically adolescent behaviors to test them on top of the long-term ADHD difficulties. For parents who are already stressed, discouraged, and angry, these new behaviors, although normal and predictable developmentally, can be the last straw. Many parents at this stage of their family's life are simply overwhelmed and have given up trying to maintain control as parents. In these chaotic situations the marital relationship has been pushed aside for many years. These parents report that they have had too much conflict with one another over parenting to be trusting, loving, or sexual with each other. Marital therapy with parents of ADHD adolescents often reveals patterns of either high levels of conflict and animosity or equally high levels of distance and avoidance. The focus of early interventions with ADHD families, as we have described, is toward stabilization of the family's overall functioning by normalizing the role of the ADHD child or adolescent in the family and diffusing the scapegoating patterns for both parents and siblings. We have found that it is not realistic for the therapist to attempt to work clinically with the parents' marital relationship until the family's general chaos has been addressed and lessened. Otherwise, efforts to focus on the marital dynamics will be sabotaged and diverted by the overwhelming parental and family conflicts. Once some stabilization has occurred, however, the parents are now more available emotionally and pragmatically to begin to focus on their own personal relationship.

Marital therapy at this stage often begins with a session or two in which spouses are asked to recall how they met and why they were attracted to one another. Many partners will have lost touch with these early events and images, particularly with the romantic qualities of their former lives. Since most early mate selection carries an element of romantic idealization, it is fairly safe to ask even the unhappiest of couples to recall their early attraction. The therapist who starts with these early dynamics, particularly if he or she does in a casual or playful manner, relieves the spouses of their ever-present stress regarding parenting issues, opens a new window for them to look back upon their life together, and reminds them of what they have lost over the years. Often at this point partners tearfully share with one another their sense of loss and despair. Spouses now verbalize the pain they feel over multiple losses: companionship, of their "best friend," intimacy, a sexual partner, a fun partner, and simply the privacy or time to be alone together.

We find that many of these spouses feel abandoned by their partners. Sometimes the wife feels that the husband has abandoned her to become a workaholic so that he is unavailable to her to help with parenting or household chores. Or, the husband may feel that the wife has abandoned him to become totally absorbed in the caretaking tasks of motherhood. Both share their long-term struggles with each other and their exhaustion with their ADHD adolescent's problems. These mutual reflections can dramatically reconnect a couple emotionally by calling their attention to their early attraction and bonding. Indeed, this important reconnection can often be accomplished in the initial marital session—unless the level of animosity has reached such significant proportions that one or both spouses is/are contemplating divorce.

The experience of reconnecting emotionally opens the door clinically for defining clearer and firmer boundaries around their spousal subsystem. This involves discussions of how to create privacy and time together for dates, trips, and sexual encounters with one another. These bonding experiences in the marital therapy reinforce for the couple their need to prioritize their own personal and relationship needs. This emotional shift brings about a healthy reduction in their investment in parenting and a natural redefinition of their roles as parents.

Most parents of ADHD adolescents benefit from more objectivity—not necessarily more distance—in coping with their children, including the non-ADHD children. The spouses need to begin talking about parenting as a team, making firmer and more consistent decisions, and supporting rather than sabotaging one another. While these issues of coparenting were identified with the parents in the earliest sessions and reinforced throughout therapy, their abilities to embrace and enact these roles may not occur until the distance and animosity in the marital relationship has subsided. Coparenting is important—if not essential—with ADHD adolescents, whose ability to argue, debate, manipulate, and intimidate is much more dramatic than an ADHD child's. Gradually increased parenting skills will reduce the adolescent's ability to "divide and conquer" by playing one parent against the other. These skills will also serve the parents well in parenting other children in the home and returning stability to the family's overall functioning. Couples who have an underlying attachment that has not been too severely damaged over the years can make substantial, even dramatic, changes in these areas during marital therapy over just four to six sessions.

It is important to point out that in families where the spouses have made dramatic changes, particularly in defining and enforcing clearer boundaries with all of their children, we often hear about (and observe for ourselves) a period of reactivity by the non-ADHD children that takes the form of angry outbursts at home or at school. Consistent with the principle of circularity that characterizes family systems, the non-ADHD siblings have become used to having immediate and unencumbered access to both parents, even while feeling "left out" due to the focus on their ADHD sibling. Now when they hear their parents saying that they can no longer drop everything and take them to their friend's house or to the mall, or when they see their parents going out on a date or planning a trip together, they often feel that they are losing what limited attention they had been able to expect from their parents. Some of these siblings tell us they wish that we had not "messed up their family" and that they feel like they are losing their parents. These dynamics can be managed therapeutically in the context of additional family sessions by structuring the parents' new need for privacy in a way that ensures the children quality time with one or both parents.

An exception to some of the above parental and marital dynamics occurs when one of the spouses also has ADHD. This, of course, adds another layer of complicated clinical symptoms and dynamics to the parent–child and marital interactions. We will discuss this area in the next chapter on adults. Another exception may occur with couples who are considering divorce; in such case, marital therapy may simply be too late. Even with the changes that they experience with their ADHD adolescent and in the family as a whole, the long-term conflict may have eroded their bonding too significantly to repair. Thus the role of marital therapy at this point is to help the spouses clearly and openly articulate their intentions to leave the relationship and help them make a plan for separation or divorce that will be responsive to the needs of their children (see Everett & Volgy-Everett, 1994).

8

Developing Therapeutic Interventions for Adults with ADHD and Their Families

Most ADHD adults do not seek treatment directly: they are identified primarily in other contexts. Despite increased public awareness regarding ADHD in adults, it has been our experience, supported informally by anecdotal reports from other professionals, that very few ADHD adults actually refer themselves or seek consultation regarding their symptoms. We estimate that as many as 70% of the adults we have identified with ADHD were discovered in the course of our evaluations of their ADHD offspring. Perhaps another 20% were diagnosed with ADHD in the course of ongoing therapy for other symptoms or problems, such as depression, substance abuse, anxiety, occupational failure, or marital conflict. About 5% per cent were brought to therapy by a spouse who had read about ADHD and suspected that her or his partner had the disorder. Another 5% were referred to us by physicians, psychiatrists, or other therapists who know that we work with ADHD clients in our practices.

Many ADHD adults, when they learn of their child's ADHD symptoms, acknowledge openly, and occasionally tearfully, that they have struggled most of their lives with similar difficulties. Some of these adults have told us, in essence, "I always knew that he [the son] was just like me, but I never knew there was a name for our problem," or "I knew he was doing all of the things that got me into trouble when I was his age, but I hoped it would get better." Regarding the latter type of remark, occasionally a frustrated wife (or husband) will remark sarcastically, "Well, it never got better for you!"

Many undiagnosed ADHD adults respond cautiously or resistantly when the symptoms are explained to them. Some use the similarity of behaviors and experiences that they see in their child as a defense to justify their own earlier school failures or to deny their present symptomatic behaviors. These adults may have considerable resistance to accepting the ADHD diagnosis in their child because it would mean admitting that they have the disorder themselves. Indeed, more often it is the non-ADHD spouse who is quick to offer her (or his) own diagnosis of ADHD for the partner. Describing years of struggles and frustrations, the spouse reports her or his pent-up feelings using descriptors such as *reactive, restless, irritable, distractible, forgetful, unable to relax or play,* and *impatient with the children.*

The evaluation of an undiagnosed ADHD adult is somewhat more variable than the evaluation of children and adolescents. Psychoeducational testing is central to the overall evaluation and development of a realistic treatment plan for children and adolescents because they are in their formative years and actively involved in the educational system. The testing data provide the therapist and educator with specific information regarding deficits that will affect their future learning and educational experiences. Since most ADHD adults are no longer in school, testing is not essential for their evaluation. Moreover, adults are more articulate and can reflect more accurately on their own symptoms, and most have a spouse who can also identify symptomatic patterns. Thus we do not believe that costly psychoeducational or psychological evaluations for ADHD adults (which may range up to $1,000) are necessary. While test data may be helpful, we have found that most adults have completed their education and their areas of difficulty appear more focused now in marital, family, social, and occupational experiences.

However, in the process of an evaluation, we may find that many ADHD adults are making plans to return to school to complete unfinished degrees or high school diplomas with new hope for success. Others had such difficult school experiences that they would never consider returning to an educational setting. Certainly, for those ADHD adults who gain renewed confidence about successfully returning to school, testing is recommended to assist them in making appropriate educational and/or career choices, as well as to qualify them for the special services that most universities now offer. For example, ADHD adults who develop proficiency on their home computers may consider becoming computer programmers and consultants. However, faced with the academic demands and mathematics required in these programs, many shy away because of the shadow of past failures, stating something like, "I flunked high school algebra three times." ADHD adults who report that they continue to be restless, to be easily bored, and to have difficulty paying attention for long periods may benefit from stimulant medications if they decide to return to school. Most junior colleges and universities now have supportive programs for students with disabilities (including ADHD), programs that did not exist when these adults were first considering further education or training in young adulthood. We often refer these recently diagnosed ADHD adults to private career counselors or similar services provided by community colleges.

ADHD may also be identified as part of a work-related referral or evaluation. An employee may be having difficulty relating to supervisors and colleagues or completing work assignments in a timely fashion. Testing may be recommended in this context, and in most cases would be supported by the employer who wants the worker to remain with the company. The test results would not only confirm the ADHD diagnosis but would provide his or her employer with useful information regarding the employee's strengths and weaknesses in terms of the job description. (We will discuss a case regarding these issues later in this chapter.)

As is the case with children and adolescents, the evaluation of ADHD in adults may be complicated by the presence of a variety of comorbid symptoms and disorders. Many nondiagnosed ADHD adults who are in therapy may have already been diagnosed with a variety of other psychiatric disorders; in some instances these comorbid disorders mask the ADHD symptoms. More commonly these other symptoms become the primary focus of treatment and no consideration is given to ADHD factors. Barkley and Murphy (1993) cautions clinicians not to discount the presence of ADHD when other disorders are present, stating that the practice of diagnosing ADHD in adults only when no other disorders are present is "illogical" and "overly restrictive." Many studies have confirmed that even where no prior or comorbid psychiatric diagnoses exist for ADHD adults, the ADHD adult will experience concurrent problem areas in social and family relations, marital relationships, and employment. However, the presence of a comorbid disorder's more easily recognizable symptoms may obscure the underlying ADHD symptoms.

The clinical evaluation of ADHD adults should include the same thorough history taking (developmental, social, and educational) that we have recommended for children and adolescents (Table 8.1). It should also include a careful review of roles and performances in social and work settings. We utilize two additional sources of information to gain data and corroborate our diagnostic impressions. The first source is the ADHD adult's spouse, who can offer clear confirmation

TABLE 8.1. Historical Information for Adult ADHD Diagnosis

1. Early childhood medical and developmental history
2. Preschool childhood experiences with parents, siblings, and peers
3. Educational history: grade school, middle school, high school, college
4. Social history throughout childhood, adolescence, and young adulthood
5. Adult social interaction patterns
6. Adult relationship patterns
7. Adult parenting roles
8. Adult occupational history and roles

of everyday behaviors. The second source is a personal or telephone consultation with the ADHD adult's parents, or other family-of-origin members, such as siblings, who can provide us with valuable information about childhood and adolescent behaviors.

The spouse of an ADHD partner can provide a descriptive array of everyday symptoms for the therapist. A parent can offer her or his impressions of the adult child's early developmental experiences and add information about early behavioral and educational experiences that many adults who struggled during those years might have forgotten (or repressed). Most parents and family-of-origin members are very willing to offer information and reflections. (We will discuss the educational and therapeutic benefits of these consultations below.) We have conducted telephone consultations for ADHD adults with their parents, siblings, grandparents, foster parents, adoptive parents, aunts and uncles, and in one case a former high school girlfriend. We have also been sent report cards and samples of the ADHD adult's early school work by parents who hoped that these documents might assist our evaluation.

Most adults are eager to understand this often unexplained and frustrating part of their life experience, and therefore willing to involve family-of-origin members. They are also willing to read about ADHD. During this evaluation period we often suggest that *both* spouses read Hallowell and Ratey's (1994) book and discuss their impressions. It is important to request that *both* spouses participate in the reading assignment because many ADHD adults simply do not enjoy reading: without the support and expectations of their partner, they will never complete the suggested books.

We have found that Hallowell and Ratey's book has just the right balance of technical and medical information. Moreover, the book's many brief reports of personal experiences with ADHD enable undiagnosed ADHD adults to identify immediately with the symptomatic patterns. Many previously undiagnosed adults return for an appointment after reading this book and announce that the book was "written about me" or "described my life perfectly." One adult came into the office carrying the book, with a smile on his face, and stated: "You might as well put my picture on the cover of this book—it's all about me." Sometimes, too, it is the non-ADHD spouse who returns after reading the book, excited and elated by an objective and comprehensive description of how her or his spouse behaves.

The range of clinical interventions and treatment sequences that we outlined for working with ADHD children and adolescents cannot be as clearly defined for adults. Clinical work with the ADHD adult tends to focus on individual and marital therapy, with family and intergenerational issues identified at appropriate times. Some ADHD adults respond better to individual sessions at first; for others, the marital sessions are the most productive. For many, we find that we can blend individual and conjoint sessions in an alternating week format. In addition, the three roles for the therapist previously described— psychoeducation, advocacy, and therapy—also take on somewhat different aspects in working with ADHD adults.

EVALUATING ADULTS WITH ADHD

In our work the early phases of evaluation and discussion of ADHD usually occur in the context of a marital interview. A few adults do request individual sessions first to learn more about their ADHD because they are embarrassed by their condition, want to avoid confrontations with their spouse, or are considering divorce. However, in most cases the early interviews are conducted with both spouses present.

Working with the marital dyad to determine a clinical evaluation of one spouse may seem odd and uncomfortable to therapists who have been trained to complete evaluations in the privacy of individual interviews. Our strong preference for this format is based on our clinical experience that many ADHD adults are not accurate or effective reporters of their own long-term behavioral or historical patterns and roles, and often do not have a realistic sense of how their symptomatic behaviors have impacted their family and social relationships. We have also observed that many of these adults are incapable of accurately remembering and reporting information about individual therapy sessions to their spouses.

Throughout the early evaluation period and later during marital therapy, we solicit the support of the partner both as a consultant and a participant in therapy. Therefore, we need this partner to hear the same information and diagnostic details that we communicate to the ADHD spouse. Of course, the first underlying therapeutic goal is to assign a name to the long-term patterns that both partners have suffered from and thereby provide them with a sense of relief and hope for the future. We give them a reading list of ADHD resources that we have found specifically helpful for adults (see Appendix 6.1 in Chapter 6, page 194) as well as various articles and handouts. However, the majority of ADHD adults will not spend much time (if any) reading these materials. It is important for the therapist to understand that this is not necessarily an expression of resistance to therapy, as might be concluded when a patient fails to read information provided to her or him on communication, but is simply an extension of the ADHD adult's lifelong struggles with attention, reading, and memory. The spouse may be the only one to read the materials. We have found that a brief and straightforward checklist format is the most effective tool for gaining an immediate response. We use a checklist that identifies a broad range of ADHD symptoms from a variety of sources (see Table 2.4). We give each spouse a copy of this checklist and ask each of them to independently check the items that apply before comparing notes. There is rarely congruence between the items checked by the ADHD spouse and the non-ADHD partner.

Early in the evaluation we want to link the adult's ADHD symptoms with the broader issues of marital communication, parenting, and occupational roles. Many couples struggling in their relationship will quickly jump into identifying their many conflicted areas. However, we try to maintain a balance here, so that the diagnostic and psychoeducational information can also have an impact. *A premature focus on marital or family conflict will diffuse the clarity of the ADHD diagnosis.* Unlike the procedure in more general marital therapy, in therapy for ADHD a specific treatment plan for improving the ADHD symptoms must be established first, preceding the broader marital and family treatment plan. If the ADHD symptoms do not improve, the marital therapy will often get bogged down in unresolvable layers of past and current conflicts.

We are comfortable giving an ADHD diagnosis for most adults based on a careful review of their personal and educational histories (confirmed and elaborated, where possible, by spouse and/or family-of-origin members), their current behaviors and interactions (confirmed by a spouse or partner), their overall educational and occupational experiences, and their self-report of long-term and present symptom patterns. Of course, the therapist may also refer to the DSM-IV (American Psychiatric Association, 1994) diagnostic criteria, where (see discussion in Chapter 2) at least six of the nine criteria in either the inattentive or the hyperactive–impulsive categories are required to justify the diagnosis.

We have never been comfortable relying entirely on these formal DSM criteria. We view these criteria as a baseline for the diagnosis, but we add much more behavioral and familial data to the clinical picture. This is why we routinely consult with spouses and family-of-origin members. In our clinical files at the initial interview we have a one-page listing of the DSM-IV (American Psychiatric Association, 1994) criteria that we use as a private checklist in the early interviews. We want to be able to support our diagnosis technically, but we are never satisfied with just these data. We certainly make testing available for these adults if they wish to pursue it, but most do not. Some adults who are intrigued with the disorder and its meaning for them, and who can afford to pay for private testing, will do so to satisfy their own curiosity. If one's practice is populated by middle-income patients, however, who rely on managed care services, the possibility of insurance reimbursement for testing may be quite limited.

After the diagnosis has been confirmed, and if there are children 8 years and older in the family, we frequently schedule a family session with the children and parents in order to support the ADHD parent while she or he explains the ADHD diagnosis. We believe that it is an important healing step for the recently diagnosed ADHD parent to explain what she or he has learned about the disorder to her or his children. Our role in these sessions is to answer questions, clarify more technical issues, and help to explain to the children how the disorder has affected their ADHD parent's interaction with them over the years. We will often encourage the ADHD parent to share with her or his children memories about and reflections on her or his own early school and growing-up experiences now that she or he understands them better in light of the ADHD diagnosis. As with most psychoeducational interventions, the underlying therapeutic goal here is to increase acceptance of the disorder and to provide hope for successful treatment outcomes.

Most children are responsive to this initial family meeting, which also sets the stage for future family therapy sessions. Many parents tell us that they are surprised by the immediate improvement in their children's behaviors and attitudes following this first family meeting. We suspect that this occurs so rapidly because (1) the children are pleased that their parent is seeking help, (2) they are relieved to discover an explanation for some of the difficulties they have experienced with their ADHD parent, and (3) they have hope for positive change.

We have also conducted similar meetings with ADHD adults' families-of-origin members. Often we meet with the parents of the

ADHD adult who are eager to know more about the disorder, and who may also be looking for relief from an underlying guilt they may have carried for years regarding their inadequacy or failure as a parent to this child. We have listened to many tearful parents of ADHD adult children express profound relief upon learning that there really was something wrong with their child. Many parents talk about having had early "instincts" or "intuition" that something was wrong with their child, and express frustration about never being able to convince the school or doctors about their suspicions. One mother, a retired teacher in her mid-60s, cried and said, "You don't know how relieved I am that my son is getting help. Now I can let go of all of the bad feelings that I never did enough or somehow made things worse for him. Thank you."

In another case, some months after an ADHD adult had been diagnosed, had been medicated, and had begun to experience positive changes in his marriage and with his children, one of the authors (CAE) received a call from the patient asking if the author would be willing to talk to his father by phone. He would not say exactly what the father wanted, but noted that the author would be "amused." Several days later the father called. He was a retired naval officer with a daughter and three other sons scattered around the country. He said he was so impressed by the changes in his ADHD son over the past couple of months that he wanted to pay to fly his daughter, her husband, and his three sons and their spouses to Tucson and then pay for as many hours of family therapy as was needed to repair the "abusive and negative" experiences to which his son had been subjected in the family. He also asked for a preliminary evaluation to determine whether his daughter and possibly a grandchild might also have ADHD. The author told the father that it was not necessary to bring all of these family members to Tucson for evaluations and offered referrals in their respective communities. However, it was agreed that the parents and several of the siblings, without spouses, would come for a weekend to participate in several family-of-origin sessions to bring closure to past disputes and initiate a healing process in their relationships.

ADVOCACY ISSUES FOR THE ADULT WITH ADHD

As with children and adolescents, the therapist can often play an important role as an advocate for ADHD adults. However, the advocacy role may involve broader issues with adults. After an adult receives an ADHD diagnosis, she or he often needs help to explain and seek support for the disorder at many points in her or his family, social, and occupational network. Certainly, the psychoeducational family meeting that we described, as well as the occasional family-of-origin meetings, provide an opportunity for the therapist to serve as an advocate with family members for the ADHD adult. In performing this role, it is important for the therapist to understand that advocacy does not mean defending or justifying harmful or hurtful behaviors. If the therapist oversteps this sensitive line, she or he will risk alienating both spouse and children who may have experienced years of tumultuous interactions with the ADHD adult. The advocacy for the therapist should be clearly focused on providing information and explanations for other family members.

The more dramatic advocacy role with ADHD adults often occurs in their work settings. Many ADHD adults have found comfortable and stable work environments. Many have also learned to create their own accommodations in the types of work they have sought and the settings in which they found they could function best. In fact, many ADHD adults who learn to utilize their unlabeled ability of hyperfocusing become quite successful if they are able to find and secure compatible work settings. A study by Banks and associates (1995) of medical students who were unsuccessful in medical school and of recently graduated physicians who failed their licensing exams reported that 78% had either a learning disorder or ADHD, yet their ability to compensate had allowed them to reach a high level of education, failing only "in the last stretch." We have worked with several ADHD, hyperactive–impulsive type, physicians who were effective and comfortable in emergency medical settings but who reported being bored and unchallenged in office practices. Several of these physicians had changed practice settings frequently. Of the ones who did not find a role in emergency settings, one settled into an educational setting that was more stimulating for him. Others moved from their office practices to public health or low-income community clinics. All had difficulties in their marital and family lives. None was referred because of suspected ADHD. However, one acknowledged that he had secretly been taking Ritalin samples for 5 years to calm himself during the day (he never considered the ADHD diagnosis—he just found that Ritalin worked). The majority of the other physicians were referred either due to their children's difficulties and/or chronic marital problems. For many of these physicians, receiving the diagnosis and learning about the disorder was enough to help them begin to find their own ways of focusing, restructuring their time, and developing stimulating experiences with their spouses and children.

This role of advocacy for ADHD adults in their work settings is typically psychoeducational in nature. For ADHD adults who identify chronic struggles and difficulties in occupational settings, the therapist can perform a helpful role by writing a carefully worded letter to the patient's manager or supervisor explaining the ADHD diagnosis, the symptoms in general, disability aspects, the legal requirements for accommodations with regard to this type of disability, and a list of potential accommodation for the particular employee (similar to the list one prepare for 504 conferences in school settings). Large companies typically have policies regarding disabilities, but these policies may never have been interpreted for ADHD employees.

Sometimes employers will ask for a meeting with the employee and the therapist. In other situations the patient asks the employer for such a meeting. In certain circumstances we ourselves recommend a meeting, for example, if we feel that the employee's future employment is in jeopardy, or if she or he appears to be struggling or feels harassed by supervisors. That was the situation in the following case.

One of the authors (CAE) had been working for over 6 months with a single man who had been diagnosed previously with learning disabilities and ADHD. He was originally referred by a psychiatric facility following hospitalization for severe depression. The depression had developed after he had been fired from his third job in 3 years. Most of his prior employment settings had involved menial physical labor. His history indicated that he was dyslexic and somewhat slow in processing auditory information, particularly in conversations. Some of his family and former employers thought that he might be retarded. Even the intake counselor at the hospital had indicated in her admission notes the possibility of retardation.

He had been raised on a farm in the Midwest and had graduated from a small high school with low to average grades. He said that his brothers all performed much better in school than he. He had never been evaluated for school problems and had never even heard of ADHD. His family members, including his father, often called him "stupid" or "retard"—designations he continued to apply to himself. He said that his mother was the only one in his family who was supportive and did not pick on him.

Before his discharge from the hospital he had been given a full range of psychological tests. To everyone's amazement at the hospital, even the testing psychologist, his Full-Scale WAIS score was 122.

He liked his present job as a handyman for a small apartment complex. Historically, his depressive symptoms seemed to follow his relative success or failure in a work setting. He did not report any memory of depression during his childhood or adolescence. His father was deceased, his mother was in a nursing home, and he was not close to his siblings, so there were no options to gain corroborative early data. He did report that he had been an offensive lineman on the high school football team and, as he put it, "hung out with the jocks," but never felt accepted or that he "fit in." He had not dated in high school and had only been out with three women as an adult.

His present employers were often demanding and critical, particularly with regard to his inability to remember instructions and assignments. Whenever he was reprimanded by his employers, he would become sullen and withdrawn, telling himself that he really was stupid. When the diagnosis of ADHD, inattentive type, with LD was explained to him, he was amazed, exclaiming to the therapist, "You mean, I'm really not stupid?" Initially the therapist worked with him on practical skills to compensate for his attention difficulties and poor short-term memory. He began to make lists of daily tasks, but the lists were insufficient and his employers were still impatient with him. Driven to Distraction (Hallowell & Ratey, 1994) was recommended to him, but he could only read a few pages at a time. He did leave it for one of his employers to read, to no avail. He was medicated with Ritalin, but experienced only minor improvement. He was able to say that he felt more focused on the job and that he did not leave as many projects unfinished. However, much more dramatic improvement occurred when an antidepressant was added.

The therapist was concerned that his job might be in jeopardy, so it was recommended that he request a meeting with the therapist and his employers at the apartment complex. The initial goal was to educate the employers about his ADHD and LD symptoms and about resources. An additional goal, if the employers were amenable, was to negotiate a clearer role definition and more reasonable expectations for him at work. The employers were responsive to the meeting and, despite their frustrations, stated that he was quite valued because he was friendly, took time to talk to the residents, and was the most popular handyman they had ever had. One of the employers, in particular, was quite surprised to learn of the employee's ADHD, even acknowledging in the meeting that he had a nephew who had struggled with ADHD. He asked the author for suggestions about books to read for himself and his sister's family.

This brief but dramatically effective meeting opened the door for clearer communication and interaction between the employee and employer and a greater understanding and appreciation of the ADHD adult's role. Many practical suggestions were accepted regarding putting requests for projects and tasks in writing and prioritizing the various items on the list. Much of the ensuing therapy for the individual focused on improving his chronically low self-esteem and helping him learn new skills and accommodations to his ADHD. He was referred to the state rehabilitation program for further evaluation for potential training in more advanced job skills.

This case demonstrates the value of the therapist's role as advocate, in this situation to educate the employer. If the therapy for this ADHD adult had proceeded without intervention in the work setting, it would have been of limited value in building confidence and self-esteem because of the patient's continued stress and failure at work. The therapist's presence in a face-to-face meeting helped the employer to understand that the patient's deficiencies reflected a disability rather than a character flaw and even to recognize the similarity to his nephew's diagnosis. Without intervention by the therapist, the patient probably would have lost his job and the therapist would have been forced to deal with another depressive episode instead of helping the patient progress toward further job training. As was true in the case described above, many newly diagnosed ADHD adults benefit from a reevaluation of their career choices. Many do consider returning to school or receiving supplemental training. Most will benefit from specialized career consultations (Nadeau, 1995). As with ADHD children and adolescents, the evaluation and diagnosis is never sufficient on its own to accomplish therapeutic change.

The therapist may also need to advocate on behalf of ADHD patients with other professionals. As we have indicated, many undiagnosed ADHD adults are in treatment for other psychiatric disorders or are referred for evaluation of these other disorders. One of the most frequently required advocacy roles is with physicians over the issue of medication, which may involve more complex medical and pharmacological issues, particularly if the patient is taking medications for other medical conditions. In these situations, the possible use of stimulant medication needs to be evaluated for interactive ramifications. As we mentioned previously, many physicians, as well as psychiatrists and other therapists, may have little information about the diagnosis and treatment of ADHD in adults, which the therapist/advocate can remedy by taking an active role.

Despite a growing volume of literature about ADHD in adults, many professionals do not consider ADHD to be an adult disorder. Often after we have evaluated an adult for ADHD and made the diagnosis, we contact other therapists already involved with either the ADHD adult or other family members to offer consultation and education regarding the disorder. Many times it is difficult to convince another therapist that the complaints heard from the wife about her husband's long-term disruptive behaviors are, indeed, symptomatic of ADHD. Occasionally, we hold joint meetings with the therapist treating the other spouse or children in much the same format as the family feedback sessions we conduct for children and adolescents. Sometimes we continue to treat the adult individually regarding the ADHD symptoms and then refer her or him back to the other therapist for marital or family sessions.

Legal and court-related issues are typically focused on helping ADHD adults understand and, if needed, access resources regarding their legal rights (Latham & Latham, 1995) and assisting them in gaining disability accommodations in their work settings. If there is no significant response to the initial contact or letter in which we explain the disability and identify the needed accommodations, we then refer the ADHD adult to a consulting attorney. Often the attorney's letter elicits an immediate positive response. However, a few cases may move toward a court hearing, in which case the therapist is often asked to write an affidavit regarding the diagnosis itself and the claimant's basis for the diagnosis, or to participate in a deposition.

We have assisted ADHD adults in other areas of legal difficulties, such as offering diagnostic opinions to parole and probation officers regarding the potential contribution of ADHD to substance abuse or domestic violence. We have also provided evaluations and ongoing therapy for ADHD individuals based on parole or probation stipulations for participation in therapy. We have assisted several divorced ADHD parents in their pursuit of custody or access to their children when it was apparent that their history of ADHD in the marriage and family was being used to strengthen a case against their parental competency.

MARITAL DYNAMICS OF COUPLES WITH ADHD

We have found that marital therapy is often the most productive therapeutic setting for working with the ADHD adult. As noted, the spouse can provide much needed corroboration of data during the early evaluation phase and can offer support during the psychoeducational stages of therapy. We have also noted the importance of treating the marital subsystem as part of the stabilization of the ADHD family, even when the ADHD member is a child or adolescent. In families where the ADHD member is a spouse, or where the spouse is one of multiple ADHD members in the nuclear system, we believe that marital therapy is often crucial to the survival of the family. In fact, many cases in which we have identified an ADHD adult have been referred initially and primarily for marital problems.

The typical areas of conflict reported by spouses, where one has ADHD, are summarized under the following categories:

1. Communication.
2. Personal intimacy, attentiveness, and sexuality.
3. Leisure time for personal activities and socializing with friends.
4. Finances and money management.
5. Parenting responsibilities.

6. Household tasks and responsibilities.
7. Work and career issues.
8. Alcohol and substance abuse.

Many of these problem areas have been present from the beginning of the relationship. Therefore, the focus of the marital therapy is on repairing and undoing the damage that has been incurred as a result of the problematic interplay of undiagnosed ADHD symptoms and "normal" marital dynamics. In many non-ADHD marital therapy cases, one can ask a couple to review their years together and identify periods when they were happier or more satisfied with one another. Unless simply mismated from the beginning, most couples can recall their early attraction to one another, romantic periods during their courtship, and early marital bonding. Some couples recall their early happiness deteriorating only after the arrival of the first or second child. Others report ups and downs throughout their marriage.

The two most striking features about ADHD marriages are that:

- There are often few happy or contented times reported over the course of the relationship by the non-ADHD spouse.
- The ADHD spouse is often surprised and oblivious to her or his partner's long-term list of complaints and unhappy feelings, as well as to the partner's degree of emotional disappointment and dissatisfaction.

The chronicity of the ADHD symptoms and their intrusion, even from courtship days, into the normal development of a marital relationship can disrupt the process of bonding and intimacy so important in anchoring a marriage. The fact that the non-ADHD spouse selected an ADHD partner, having experienced the symptoms (diagnosed or not) from the start of the relationship, raises interesting questions regarding mate selection and complementarity in the ADHD relationship. The clinical question is, What was the non-ADHD spouse attracted to in her or his courtship of the ADHD partner?

Unfortunately, no clinical literature has addressed issues of mate selection and complementarily for ADHD couples. In a discussion of general mate selection dynamics, Dicks (1967) observed that individuals have a "mutual signaling system" that helps them locate safe and comfortable prospective partners. In marital therapy, one looks at the early patterns of mate selection and the underlying complementarity during the initial assessment. The mate selection often defines the levels of emotional maturity, degrees of individuation from families of origin, and underlying expectations of marital roles, particularly for young adults in their first marriages (see Nichols & Everett, 1987).

The degree of early complementarity will determine the parameters of the couple's potential for emotional balance and ongoing patterns of communication and intimacy. For example, a young man who has trouble leaving home and differentiating from his family of origin due to underlying dependency will typically seek a partner who can play a nurturing and caretaking role in order to replicate, as much as possible, the security he has experienced in his family of origin. The prospective partner may have been an eldest sibling and caretaker of younger brothers in her family of origin, and the prospect of caretaking a somewhat dependent but safe male partner feels familiar to her. These complementary roles, simply stated, circumscribe not only the range and balance of the relationship but also characterize the couple's communication, intimacy, and future parenting roles. For such a relationship a future crisis might occur when the male "grows up" and no longer wishes or needs to be taken care of, or when the female "grows up" and no longer wishes or needs to take care of her partner. This challenge to the underlying complementarity of their relationship can threaten the survival of the marriage (see Everett & Everett, 1994; Nichols & Everett, 1987).

For ADHD couples, a complementary pattern in mate selection appears to be present with both male and female ADHD spouses, whether hyperactive–impulsive or inattentive types, and whether in first or successive marriages. The ADHD spouse typically brings into the marriage an underlying immaturity with associated emotional dependent characteristics. These are family-of-origin patterns that extend, if uninterrupted, from adolescence into adulthood. Without even considering the ADHD symptoms, the therapist would recognize that this pattern alone would tend to attract a partner who needs to play a caretaking role, either for reasons of safety or familiarity.

But the dynamics of this pattern become more dramatic when ADHD symptoms are added to the mix. A common question from therapists, as well as for non-ADHD spouses is, "Why would a perfectly healthy individual select, marry, and put up with an ADHD partner's crazy-making behaviors?" The clinical issues here are twofold:

1. The non-ADHD partner may not be as healthy or mature as perceived.
2. This partner may actually be attracted to certain aspects of the ADHD symptoms.

Non-ADHD partners may experience their own issues of low self-confidence and low self-esteem. If they grew up in a family playing the role of a caretaker to their siblings, or even to their parents, their awareness that their new partner may need (and require) caretaking is not at all uncomfortable. In fact, these roles of caretaker and pleaser are consistent with their internal image of themselves. The non-ADHD partner's relative level of emotional needs and immaturity matches, to some degree, that of her or his ADHD partner's. In fact, the comfort of this caretaking role may dominate the non-ADHD partner's early idealization of the relationship such that the underlying warning signals are not recognized.

Dicks (1967) observed that in some marriages, over time, partners may begin to resent the actual characteristics and traits that originally attracted them to one another. With regard to ADHD couples, we have found that the non-ADHD spouse is often attracted to aspects of the partner's ADHD behaviors, even though later these become irritants in the relationship. Non-ADHD partners report being attracted to the high levels of energy and intensity, the passion, and the active-oriented life style of the ADHD partner. Table 8.2 offers a comparative list we have developed that identifies some of the positives (strengths) and negatives (weaknesses) of personal traits and behaviors ADHD adults typically bring into their marital relationships. We often give this list to ADHD couples to help them objectify some of the ADHD partner's traits and reframe their long-term conflicts to see underlying positive dimensions.

The attractiveness of ADHD adults in mate selection lies in their characteristic high levels of *energy, active orientation toward life,* and

TABLE 8.2. Characteristic Strengths and Weaknesses of an ADHD Spouse in a Marital Relationship

Strengths	Weaknesses
Highly energetic	Impatient
Active orientation	Irritable
Creative	Moody
Curious	Egocentric
Enthusiastic	Intolerant of noise and confusion
Passionate	Poor communication skills
Humorous	Careless with details
Intensity (positive)	Limited capacity to manage stress
	Easily bored
	Impulsive
	Disorganized
	Intensity (negative)

broad, variable personal interests. Certainly many ADHD adults display *creativity, curiosity, enthusiasm,* and *humor.* The one quality that many non-ADHD spouses identify in their reflections about their early mate selection is their partner's *intensity*—which has both positive and negative consequences in the relationship. This characteristic may be particularly attractive to a mate whose family-of-origin caretaking experiences were anything but stimulating and dramatic. For a person from such a background, the lure of excitement and stimulating activities may constitute a forbidden—and, hence, irresistible—pursuit. Certainly, many ADHD adults display levels of intensity and passion to the extremes that are expressed in risk-taking behaviors, such as skydiving or rock climbing.

The quality of passion is often a central positive ingredient in a couple's early and continuing sexual relationship and is clearly an early attractor for the non-ADHD partner. We are no longer surprised to find that many conflicted ADHD couples continue to have intercourse frequently, despite chronic levels of anger and unhappiness. Typical comments from non-ADHD partners include: "I'm not sure why I continue to have sex with him because I am so angry and hurt—but the sex is still good and gives us some way to connect" and "I don't understand how she can be so scattered and forgetful and yet so great in bed."

The reciprocal dimension of these patterns of mate selection and complementarity is that the ADHD partners are typically comfortable with the caretaking and nurturance provided by their non-ADHD spouse. Many adults who extend the caretaking roles into their adult relationships do so because it has become a familiar, safe, and status-providing component in their identity. Part of this caretaking role is the need to please others and gain approval in personal relationships. These qualities also fuel the dysfunctional aspects of the complementarity in an ADHD marriage. The early attraction to the ADHD partner's stimulating behaviors eventually becomes an irritant to the caretaking partner, but the greater need to fulfill the pleaser role often prevents this partner from challenging these behaviors early in the relationship. Many ADHD spouses simply do not have the personal resources, insight, and social skills to observe, pay attention to, and respond to their partner's complaints, whenever they are voiced. In marital sessions, many of these ADHD spouses make what appears to be a denial or at least a naive statement: "I never knew this was a problem" or "I never knew she [he] was so unhappy." In most cases this oblivion appears to be a product of the ADHD inattentive symptoms and not simply denial. Nevertheless, this unawareness of problems can be maddening for the partner and lead to escalating conflict in their relationship. Many non-ADHD partners have said, in essence, "I finally decided that I had to yell as loud as him to get his attention" or "I started throwing and breaking things to get her attention." One spouse chronicled all of her angry feelings in a journal in their computer as a daily therapeutic exercise. The ADHD spouse came across this file and expressed amazement and shock at her history of anger and frustration with him.

Practically all ADHD couples, and particularly the non-ADHD spouses, identify the conflicts as having been present from the beginning of their relationship. For most couples the levels of conflict and the erosion of their relationship worsened gradually over the years. However, some couples will report "Things were never good from the beginning" or "Once he stopped courting me, he was like a little kid to live with." Often the developmental event that dramatically escalates the couple's level of conflict and begins to breach underlying trust in the relationship is the *pregnancy and birth of the first child.* Many ADHD couples have identified this event as *the single most identifiable turning point* in the deterioration of their relationship. Pregnancy and the birth of a first child, of course, challenges and forces rebalancing of the complementarity in *all* marriages. However, the underlying dynamics of immaturity and dependency, poor communication, and lack of bonding dramatize the struggles and imbalances that are present for ADHD couples at the time of the pregnancy. The addition of parental responsibilities on top of the ongoing marital conflicts further diminishes the couple's waning personal connection.

The well-known *pursuer–distancer* marital pattern also defines much of the interaction in ADHD couples. This clinical pattern describes the role of one partner as the *pursuer* who initiates interaction and seeks attention and responses from the partner, who responds in the complementors role of *distancer,* rarely initiating interaction and withdrawing commensurately as the pursuer pursues. In some couples this interactional pattern reflects personality traits of both spouses as well as avoidance of intimacy in an unsatisfying relationship. For some couples, however, these roles may be enacted interchangeably. For example, the husband may be pursuing for a period of time and the wife distancing, followed by a reversal of these roles.

This pursuer–distancer pattern in ADHD couples often revolves around the symptoms of inattentiveness and distractibility. Theses specific symptoms can define central themes and patterns throughout the life of a couples' relationship. The non-ADHD spouse often feels unable to get the partner's attention. This inattention may range from areas like completing household tasks, to discussing bills, to offering affection, even to saying "I love you." This lack of attention in many everyday areas of family life defines the non-ADHD spouse's role clearly as the pursuer in search of responsiveness and feedback from her or his partner. This pursuit can last for years for those with strong caretaking and approval-seeking needs. Often these non-ADHD partners believe "I can't give up." Over the course of the marriage the non-ADHD spouse may internalize the lack of attention and relational responses, feeling unworthy or unattractive to the partner. Eventually, these self-critical feelings either simmer into anger, resentment, distance, and sometimes divorce, or congeal into depression and resignation.

The familiar ADHD symptom of hyperactivity appears in many adults as a chronic and unyielding *restlessness*. It takes the following forms: an inability to sit still so that the person is always on the go, looking for things to do; trying to do too many projects at once and never finishing what was started; being irritable, reactive, and impatient with the children and spouse; never taking time to sit and talk.

The *impulsive* symptom in adult relationships leads to rash purchases and credit card charges, snap decisions about activities or jobs, and reactive comments or statements that can be critical and hurtful. The non-ADHD partners complain that their spouses are impulsive, childish, and immature; that they fail to consult with their spouses about decisions and activities; and that they are "always on edge," and excessively critical.

While inattentiveness often causes non-ADHD partners to direct their frustrations inwardly, these symptoms of restlessness and impulsivity typically elicit angry responses from both the spouse and children. In fact, these impulsive behaviors may undermine the children's respect for their ADHD parent. Table 8.3 outlines many reciprocal interactive patterns that we have observed in ADHD couples.

In some ADHD marriages the pursuer–distancer roles shift when the non-ADHD spouse gives up the pursuer role and begins to disconnect emotionally from the marriage. Occasionally the ADHD spouse, realizing that the partner is seriously withdrawing or considering divorce, may desperately assume the pursuer role. Often this effort is made in vain because the non-ADHD spouse has distanced permanently.

MARITAL THERAPY FOR COUPLES WITH ADHD

In most of the literature in the field individual therapy with ADHD adults is identified as the treatment of choice. Some clinicians go slightly beyond this to recommend "multimodal" approaches (Bem-

TABLE 8.3. Interactive Patterns in ADHD Marital Relationships

The ADHD spouse's symptoms	The partner's responses
Low self-esteem	Caretaking or irritation
Excitable	Controlling or reactive
Low frustration tolerance	Angry or punitive
Volatile moods	Cautious and guarded
Intense	Withdrawing and avoiding
Depressive/anxious	Caretaking or controlling
Controlling	Distancing or struggling for power
Impulsive	Annoyed, cautious, and controlling
Restless	Frustrated and withdrawing
Poor problem solver	Controlling and angry
Short attention span	Frustrated and discounting
Distractible	Reactive and angry
Reactive/and aggressive	Avoiding, withdrawing, and confronting
Demanding	Accommodating, angry, and resentful

porad & Zambenedetti, 1996) that start with a pharmacological intervention, move to psychoeducational work, and then introduce
psychotherapy to deal with "dysfunctional personality characteristics." Others advocate the role of support groups for ADHD adults
(Kelly, 1995). Discussions of clinical work with ADHD couples are
mentioned only in passing and secondary to other treatments of
choice. In fact, we have never seen marital therapy recommended in
the literature as a viable treatment of choice for ADHD adults.

The literature offers only indirect support for the positive role of
marital and family interventions. Barkley (1997) recommends "point of
performance treatment" approaches and critiques the many cognitive–
behavioral and skill-training approaches typically recommended for
ADHD adults. He observes that one of the reasons for the relative failure
of these approaches is that they are too far removed from the primary
settings and natural milieu in which ADHD individuals function:

> The most useful treatments will be those that are in place in the natural
> settings at the point of performance where the desired behavior is to
> occur. This immediately suggests that clinic-delivered treatments,
> such as play therapy, counseling of the child, neurofeedback, or other
> such therapies are not as likely to produce clinically significant
> improvement in ADHD, if any, in comparison to treatments under-
> taken by caregivers in natural settings at the places and time where the
> performance of the desired behavior is to occur (p. 338)

We believe that Barkley's observation effectively explains, at least in
part, why our clinical experiences with marital and family therapy have

been so successful: *we work with the patient in the milieu in which the symptoms are most active.* Even if we are working with ADHD single parents, unmarried individuals, or gay individuals, we include their present partners (and occasionally past partners) in this therapy process.

As we have indicated, marital therapy cannot be constructive until some preliminary changes have occurred with the ADHD symptoms. Some ADHD adults make immediate improvements in their most problematic symptoms and begin to change the negative impact on their families. However, the overall degree of these changes, even with greater cognitive awareness, is often slow and limited. The use of stimulant medication is certainly indicated in many cases because they are effective with approximately 50–70% of adults (Barkley, 1993). We quote this proportion to our patients and their spouses; however, our own experience is that the medications are effective, at varying levels, with 90% of our adult patients.

Just as we involve the non-ADHD spouse in the evaluation and treatment process, we also involve the spouse in the discussion regarding medication for the partner. We have found that once ADHD adults begin taking medication, many do not recognize the effects of the stimulants very quickly while others will simply resist the medication and deny that they even "need drugs." Some will discount the positive effects, despite confirmation by spouses and children, for weeks. Therefore the spouse, who obviously has a personal investment in the medication being effective, again becomes an important therapeutic ally. In fact, it is often the spouse who first calls us several days after the start of medication to tell us that the effects are "amazing" or "dramatic." Nevertheless, when we see the couple together during the next session, the ADHD spouse will often seem unaware of the changes the spouse has observed. We believe that this dynamic may result from a combination of the ADHD individual's lack of personal and behavioral insight and the individual's resistance to acknowledging being helped by medication. In other words, the positive effect of the medication represents a confirmation that the disorder really exists for the individual.

Ongoing marital therapy can proceed effectively after some success in the stabilization of the family and management of the ADHD symptoms. If the marital therapy is begun prematurely, before evidence of some change, dissatisfaction and anger from the non-ADHD partner will dominate the sessions. The marital therapy proceeds with several goals in mind:

1. Repair personal damage to partner and erosion of trust in the relationship.
2. Develop a plan for accommodations by the non-ADHD spouse.

3. Build trust, companionship, communication, and intimacy.
4. Develop a coparenting partnership.

The first goal of marital therapy is to begin repairing the damage experienced by the non-ADHD partner and the erosion of trust in the relationship. Once positive changes have occurred in the reduction of ADHD symptoms and behaviors, this task is not as difficult as it might sound—unless the non-ADHD partner has genuinely disconnected emotionally. In fact, it is important early in this marital process to ask the non-ADHD partner, typically in a joint session, whether she or he is still invested enough in the relationship to work on its repair and improvement. If the therapist receives an ambivalent or equivocal response, a separate individual session with the non-ADHD partner may be necessary to explore that ambivalence and help the partner determine her or his commitment to the marriage.

The accumulated and long-term disappointments and frustrations need to be verbalized by the non-ADHD partner in a setting where she or he feels genuinely *heard*. ADHD partners do not listen well due to their symptoms of inattention and restlessness. Many non-ADHD spouses tell us that they have felt "ignored" and "discounted" throughout their marriages. In the initial marital sessions we will ask the ADHD spouse to sit quietly and reflectively during the session to allow the partner to vent her or his frustrations and hurt. Often will we ask the ADHD spouse to sit next to us, or we will pull our chair closer to hers or his. This provides the therapist more direct contact with and control over the spouse's potential defensive reactions or inattentiveness. We may reach over and touch her or his arm or chair to reestablish the partner's reflective and listening posture. The disparity that exists between the perceptions of the ADHD and the non-ADHD spouses regarding marital conflicts and dissatisfaction typically causes avoidance, denial, and defensiveness. Payne (1994) reported that, in a controlled study of couples with and without an ADHD partner, the ADHD partner expressed more satisfaction with the relationship than did the non-ADHD partner. Certain issues or events obviously take more time to heal. Usually the greater improvements that have occurred in the ADHD partner's behaviors, with or without the medication, the easier it will be for the non-ADHD partner to be hopeful that a turning point is near and some closure is possible on their unhappy history.

A second goal of marital therapy is to focus on how the non-ADHD partner can make accommodations to the ADHD spouse's disability that also take her or his needs into account. Even with improvements from stimulant medication, many of the partner's symptoms may still be present to a lesser degree or may recur in certain situations. The non-ADHD partner needs to learn that thoughtful accommodations need not threaten the future of the marriage or undermine either partner's identity or self-worth. Sometimes these accommodations take the form of specifically planning and structuring their time and schedule together so that, for example, the ADHD spouse has freedom to pursue more active tasks or pastimes and the non-ADHD partner has built-in time to receive more attention, communication, and intimacy from the partner. As the non-ADHD spouse learns more about the disorder and can recognize certain behaviors, such as inattentiveness or restlessness, she or he can see these behaviors more objectively as symptoms rather than as personal attacks or deliberate avoidance of their relationship. This will result in more tolerance when the symptoms do recur.

Some couples are able to frame ADHD symptoms in a humorous context and even joke with one another and their children about the behaviors when they reappear. Other accommodations may involve the non-ADHD spouse putting most tasks or requests in writing, prioritizing individual or family activities, and learning to overlook some behaviors. Many ADHD spouses benefit from regular strenuous exercise, such as playing competitive tennis twice a week. ADHD spouses all benefit from separating their needs for action and engagement from their more routine responsibilities and activities with their spouse and children. Gradually many ADHD adults can teach themselves to enjoy some quiet time with both their partner and their children. They can also agree to try some activities and projects initiated by the partner or their children. They also need to learn many mundane accommodations such as "never leaving for the grocery store without a written list in hand."

The third goal of marital therapy focuses on developing a new sense of trust, companionship, communication, and intimacy between the spouses. For some couples, this goal may involve recalling and reviving earlier levels of attachment and bonding when these qualities were available freely. For other couples, this involves developing these qualities in a relationship where they may have never existed or rekindling them when they were present only briefly at the beginning. While this may seem like a difficult task clinically, partners who have spent most of their adult lives together and who have invested great energy in their struggles to be parents are often surprisingly motivated and willing to work hard on saving their relationship. Therapists who have only limited clinical experience with highly conflicted couples need to *be careful never to underestimate the subtleties of attachment, the bond of shared emotional histories, and the potential resiliency of the relation-*

ship. The non-ADHD partner's persistence and determination to stay with her or his ADHD spouse over the years should not be quickly pathologized or explained away.

Interventions to achieve these goals involve creating "dating" scenarios in which the ADHD spouse is asked to take more initiative for planning joint activities that take into consideration the interests and needs of the partner. Here the ADHD spouse's underlying restlessness and energy can be reframed by the therapist as highly useful in planning creative and exciting activities together. These might include taking joint tennis or golf lessons, hiking, and planning adventuresome and romantic weekend trips (without the children). We often encourage couples to take turns in planning dates or activities so that the non-ADHD spouse can introduce calmer or quieter activities that they might learn to enjoy together, such as attending concerts or plays or taking a class together. Often we even instruct couples at this stage to take turns picking movies so that they can learn to appreciate and accept the other's tastes. For couples with particularly busy careers and chaotic family situations, we help them establish, in writing, a schedule that protects both their time together and their individual privacy.

The therapist can challenge the couple to reverse roles, such that the ADHD spouse, typically the distancer, is asked to practice becoming the pursuer. Most of these spouses will need some coaching from both the therapist and their partners to renew this role from courtship days.

We mentioned above that the non-ADHD partner is often attracted to the sexual intensity expressed by the partner. The ADHD symptoms of intensity, hyperactivity, and even hyperfocusing are often present in the adult's level of sexual desire and pursuit. Hallowell and Ratey (1994) referred to this sexually focused intensity as "hyperfocused hypersexuality." As noted, this heightened level of sexual energy may allow couples to maintain a high frequency of sexual intercourse despite intense periods of conflict. On the other hand, some ADHD adults acknowledge that, at times, they have difficulty "paying attention" during lovemaking. As we indicated in Chapter 6, some children with ADHD experience a tactile sensitivity whereby they do not like to be touched, and even certain types of clothing are irritating to them. These children may have avoided much physical nurturing during their growing-up years. This symptom can be present and quite problematic for some ADHD adults who not only have difficulty enjoying touching during intercourse but who also are uncomfortable with nonsexual holding and cuddling. Murphy (1995) called this symptom "tactile defensiveness."

The fourth goal of marital therapy involves the development of a coparenting partnership. When positive changes in the marriage have occurred, the task of revisiting long-term conflicts over parenting is necessary. If the marital therapy stopped *before* this stage is reached, the ongoing issues that have plagued the couple over parenting would quickly sabotage progress in the marital therapy. *It is important to recognize that many of these spouses are also the parents of ADHD children.* Their relationship, as described in earlier chapters, often has been impacted negatively, diminished, by the stresses of rearing one or more ADHD children. In fact, many of these spouses' identities, personally and within the family, reflect parenting rather than marital roles. Therefore, additional psychoeducational work is helpful here to discuss appropriate parental management strategies, structure and boundary-setting in the family, and effective methods of discipline. (It is assumed that, regarding spouses who have ADHD children, appropriate treatment for them has already been provided and progress has been made in this area before marital issues are addressed.) Some of these parents feel so discouraged about their parenting experiences together that they voluntarily enroll in parenting classes. We may recommend such classes to the more frustrated and problematic parents. Of course, it is important that they participate together in such classes.

Sometimes there is a need to focus on past disputes, conflicts, and hurt feelings in the parenting history at this level of clinical work. These can be briefly discussed with a view toward moving from long-term conflicts and roles to present needs and opportunities for coparenting. The primary goal is to help the spouses create a team approach incorporating mutual consultation and decision making, and to empower them with a sense of their own resources and skills to be more successful together. If the marital therapy has made advances, the development of new coparenting roles will progress smoothly.

INDIVIDUAL THERAPY AND "COACHING" FOR ADULTS WITH ADHD

Some years ago Bowen (1978) reconceptualized the role of the family therapist as a coach who did not intervene directly but instead assisted an adult family member in exploring and understanding her or his role and experiences in the family of origin. We have noted that we limit our use of individual therapy for the ADHD adult in favor of working more with the marital relationship. However, when we do work with ADHD adults individually, we try to achieve the following goals:

1. To help them understand more fully the impact of their ADHD symptoms on their family life.
2. To help them look more broadly at how their ADHD symptoms have influenced their social and career relationships.
3. To deal with caution or resistances about medications (though this is usually accomplished more effectively in the marital sessions).
4. To deal with long-term issues of self-confidence and self-esteem.

These individual coaching sessions are always defined clearly in terms of a time frame and goals. The time frame is important as a marker to encourage the continued involvement and support of the non-ADHD partner during this period when she or he is not a direct participant. If we anticipate working on several of the above issues with the ADHD adult, each of which may take four or more sessions, we may see them individually for two consecutive private sessions followed by one or two marital sessions. In our opinion, *it is a mistake clinically to continue seeing the ADHD individual for a month or more without including the spouse because it diminishes the importance of the spousal role and can result in resentment toward the therapist.*

Beyond these issues, individual time with the ADHD spouse may be spent in coaching. This simply means that we are not exploring history or dynamics but advising the patient about changing behaviors that have caused ongoing difficulties. We have found that it is helpful to approach this role in a casual and often humorous or playful manner. It is also effective if the therapist can provide creative and even unexpected tasks or assignments. Sometimes we make these tasks "secrets" shared only by the therapist and the ADHD adult. Occasionally we put these "secrets" in the context of surprising the partner with new and unexpected behaviors. We usually begin with the problematic behaviors that have been identified in the marital sessions. This is a practical and straightforward approach.

For example, one spouse may have said in a marital session that she always wished that her husband (ADHD) could sit and talk to her on Saturday evenings when she was getting dressed and ready to go out with him, instead of pacing the house and harassing her about how much time she was taking. For the therapist to be effective, coaching needs to be more than simply offering practical advice. It should involve stretching the ADHD spouse's boundaries and the limits of his or her experiences, rather than just focusing on a specific behavior. To simply tell this particular ADHD spouse to sit in the living room and leave his wife alone or to sit in the bedroom quietly and listen to her talk while she dresses would not have any impact toward broader change.

In this case, the ADHD spouse rarely slowed down enough to read, much less sit patiently for a conversation, when he was ready to leave for an activity. So in the coaching session the week before their Saturday night date, the ADHD spouse was asked to select magazines (Don't begin with books!) that he might enjoy browsing through. He picked fishing magazines because he had done some fishing with his father when he was growing up (although he had never taken his own sons fishing). He was asked to buy four or five magazines before Saturday afternoon and to find a time, without announcing his intentions to anyone, to sit in a comfortable chair in the living room. He was asked to casually look through the magazines for about an hour, thereby giving family members the opportunity to pass by and wonder what he was doing. (The instruction not to announce his plan or explain his behavior is intended to interject an aspect of play and surprise into the scenario and should be included in similar interventions.) In addition, he was asked to delay getting ready himself for their evening out until after his wife had already begun so that he would not finish so soon. Furthermore, the therapist told him, that when he was ready to leave, he was to sit on the side of the bed petting his wife's poodle, which he disliked and described as neurotic and wimpy, while listening to his wife.

Occasionally it takes some ADHD spouses, particularly husbands, weeks to talk themselves into trying these types of changes. This husband knew how unhappy his wife and children were with him, so he was willing to try anything. Even before the couple's scheduled joint session the following week, the wife called on Monday morning with the question: "What on earth did you do to him? The children ran to get me Saturday afternoon because they couldn't believe it when they asked their father why he was sitting in the chair and he said he was just reading some fishing magazines. When he sat on the bed with my dog, I thought I would die—I couldn't even concentrate on getting ready. We even had to go back to the house because I forgot my purse!"

The husband was pleased with himself because he had surprised everyone (an important therapeutic ingredient to effective coaching)—which, of course, added an underlying element of stimulation. The amazement and positive feedback he received from everyone in the family gave him additional satisfaction. However, he had great difficulty understanding why his sitting on the bed with the dog had made his wife so loving and sexually responsive that night. Several months later he took his sons on a two-day fishing trip to a nearby lake for the first time.

Other aspects of coaching are not always as dramatic. Some focus on practical issues for the ADHD adult, such as writing down all important tasks and requests, prioritizing activities, working on personal organization of time and belongings, learning to engage in less active pursuits with spouse and children, and asking the children what they would like to do instead of always being the one to set the agenda. Coaching also focuses on career issues. Many of the practical skills learned in the home setting can be readily applied to their work setting: for example, writing things down to remember, improving organizational and time management skills, and using more computer resources for structuring projects and scheduling. We often refer the ADHD adult to practical, how-to books such as Nadeau's (1997) *ADD in the Workplace* and Weiss's (1994) *The Attention Deficit Disorder in Adults Workbook*. Both of these books offer a variety of practical suggestions and outlines to aid the ADHD adult in everyday functioning.

Individual time for an ADHD adult, whether it is focused on therapeutic or coaching activities, can be helpful, but it is important for the therapist to keep these sessions balanced with the ongoing marital and family sessions. Sometimes we conduct the individual sessions concurrently with the other sessions, sometimes we alternate them. However, the progress that occurs in the individual sessions must be intentionally integrated with the ongoing issues in the marital and family contexts. It is important that family members support the ADHD adult's progress, as occurred in the case example presented above. If developments in both the individual and family work are not coordinated and reinforced, progress will diminish and individual behavioral changes may even be sabotaged, unwittingly, by family members.

FAMILY THERAPY FOR ADULTS WITH ADHD

About two-thirds of our clinical time with ADHD adults is spent in marital therapy. The remaining one-third of time is divided between the individual/coaching sessions for the adult and direct family therapy. When we feel that we have made significant changes in the interactional patterns of the spouses, we begin to schedule family sessions involving the children. If the children are under 8 years old, these sessions may not be as necessary because the positive changes in the ADHD parent's behaviors and in the marriage will be sufficient to alter the overall family dynamics. However, older children need to confirm and discuss the changes made by their ADHD parent, as well as express and vent, as did their non-ADHD parent, their frustrations or hurt in living with their ADHD parent. These children also need to experience and recognize in the family sessions the improvement and changes the parents have made toward coparenting. The children will see less conflict, less fighting, and less sabotaging between their parents, but they also may experience their parents as firmer, more disciplined, and more united in their handling of everyday issues in the home. In these family sessions the therapist needs to reinforce and reempower the parents in their new roles as well as deal with any

potential backlash from the children, who may feel they are being punished or even rejected by the changes that their "new" parents are
making.

We have observed that most children appreciate these changes
and express relief about the family's improved functioning. Some may
express concern that their non-ADHD parent is now less available, or
does not agree with them as much, or is more restrictive. These
changes, perceived by the children, are typically blamed on the ADHD
parent. The therapist needs to support the newly defined coparenting
team and help the children understand that more structure and organization will benefit the family's life experiences. The ADHD parent
needs to express to her or his children the desire and plan to be more
involved in their lives.

Throughout these family sessions the therapist also needs to support the parents' need for boundaries and privacy to protect and nurture their own relationship. In family situations in which the children
are particularly resistant to these changes, the therapist can meet with
the siblings as a group to give them support, challenge their
resistances to the changes, and therapeutically encourage their support
of their parents.

*In one particularly resistant and angry sibling group of three young adoles-
cents, the therapist (CAE) finally told them, during a sibling session, that he
was going to reveal a "secret" to them. He said that their parents were very
close to getting a divorce and that they needed to "back off" and give their parents some room to be together so that their marriage would survive. This was
a calculated "strategic" message. The therapist had previously discussed the
children's resistance with the parents and told them what he was going to say.
The parents had actually made good progress in the marital therapy, but were
struggling to implement and have the changes accepted by their children.
They had seriously considered divorce several months earlier before they had
entered therapy. This message to the adolescents carried an element of truth,
while adding a dimension of urgency and crisis to get their attention. The
request was for them to take additional responsibility for their own behaviors.
Toward the end of this session considerable emotions were expressed—anger
at their ADHD parent, tearful sadness over never having felt secure as a family.*

*Such an intervention, while dramatizing the truth, quickly challenges
control dynamics in the family. Of course, the intervention would not be as
appropriate for a family with younger children. No further sessions with the
children were necessary. In fact, in a later family follow-up session, one of the
adolescents remarked how he had cautioned his brother several times after
their session with the therapist not to give his parents a hard time. So the adolescents were able to assume some responsibility for changing their own*

behaviors and dynamics in the family. As the children supported the thera-
pist's request to allow their parents more time and privacy, the parents were
able to find some special time together that quickly improved their communi-
cation and intimacy.

As discussed in earlier chapters, many families will have multiple ADHD members—perhaps a father and two children, even an uncle or grandparent. In these situations, while the clinical goals for the family remain the same, the complexity of the interactive issues increase several fold. However, the family therapy approaches that we have outlined with ADHD children and adolescents is incorporated into the family sessions with an ADHD parent. We believe that the clinical sequence of preceding from evaluation and diagnosis of ADHD in the children and/or adults, to offering psychoeducational and medical interventions, to working with the parents on better management and structure in the family, to focusing on repairing and enhancing the marital relationship, to providing advocacy and coaching when needed, to engaging all of the family members in joint sessions to develop new communication and roles will be effective in families where either one child or multiple members have ADHD.

References

Abikoff, H., Ganeles, D., Reiter, G., & Blum, C. (1988). Cognitive training in academically deficient ADDH boys receiving stimulant medication. *Journal of Abnormal Child Psychology, 16*, 411–432.

Achenbach, T. (1991). *Child Behavior Checklist.* Burlington: University of Vermont.

Ackerman, N. W. (1958). *The psychodynamics of family life.* New York: Grune & Stratton.

American Academy of Pediatrics. (1996). *Diagnostic and statistical manual for primary care, child and adolescent version.* Elk Grove, IL: Author.

American Psychiatric Association. (1968). *Diagnostic and statistical manual of mental disorders* (2nd ed.). Washington, DC: Author.

American Psychiatric Association. (1980). *Diagnostic and statistical manual of mental disorders* (3rd ed.). Washington, DC: Author.

American Psychiatric Association. (1987). *Diagnostic and statistical manual of mental disorders* (3rd ed., rev.). Washington, DC: Author.

American Psychiatric Association. (1994). *Diagnostic and statistical manual of mental disorders* (4th ed.). Washington, DC: Author.

Anastopoulos, A. (1996). Facilitating parental understanding and management of attention-deficit/hyperactivity disorder. In M. Reinecke, F. Dattilio, & A. Freeman (Eds.), *Cognitive therapy with children and adolescents* (pp. 327–343). New York: Guilford Press.

Anastopoulos, A., Guevremont, D., Shelton, T., & DuPaul, G. (1992). Parenting stress among families of children with attention deficit hyperactivity disorder. *Journal of Abnormal Child Psychology, 20*, 503–520.

Anastopoulos, A., Shelton, T., DuPaul, G., & Guevremont, D. (1993). Parent training for attention-deficit hyperactivity disorder: Its impact on parent functioning. *Journal of Abnormal Child Psychology, 21*, 581–596.

Angold, A., & Costello, E. J. (1993). Depressive comorbidity in children and adolescents: Empirical, theoretical, and methodological issues. *American Journal of Psychiatry, 150*, 1771–1779.

Applegate, B., Lahey, B., Hart, E., Waldman, I., Biederman, J., Hynd, G., Barkley, R. A., Ollendick, T., Frick, P., Greenhill, L., McBurnett, K., Newcorn, J.,

Kerdyk, L., Garfindel, B., & Shaffer, D. (1997). *Journal of the American Academy of Child and Adolescent Psychiatry, 36,* 1211–1221.

Arnold, L., & Jensen, P. (1995). Attention-deficit disorders. In H. Kaplan & B. Sadock (Eds.), *Comprehensive textbook of psychiatry* (6th ed., Vol. 2, pp. 2295–2310). Baltimore: Williams & Wilkins.

Baker, D., & McCal, K. (1995). Parenting stress in parents of children with attention-deficit hyperactivity disorder and parents of children with learning disabilities. *Journal of Child and Family Studies, 4,* 57–68.

Baldwin, K., Brown, R., & Milan, M. (1995). Predictors of stress in caregivers of attention deficit hyperactivity disordered children. *American Journal of Family Therapy, 23,* 149–160.

Ball, J. D., & Koloian, B. (1995). Sleep patterns among ADHD children. *Clinical Psychology Review, 15,* 681–691.

Banks, S., Guyer, B., & Guyer, K. (1995). A study of medical students and physicians referred for learning disabilities. *Annals of Dyslexia, 45,* 233–245.

Bar-Josef, H., Mester, R., & Rothenberg, M. (1995). Delayed detection of attention deficit disorder: A research study. *International Journal of Adolescent Medicine and Health, 8,* 53–64.

Barkley, R. A. (1977). A review of stimulant drug research with hyperactive children. *Journal of Child Psychology and Psychiatry, 18,* 137–165.

Barkley, R. A. (1990a). *Attention-deficit hyperactivity disorder: A handbook for diagnosis and treatment.* New York: Guilford Press.

Barkley, R. A. (1990b). Comprehensive evaluation of attention deficit disorder with and without hyperactivity as defined by research criteria. *Journal of Consulting and Clinical Psychology, 58,* 775–789.

Barkley, R. A. (1991). *Attention-deficit hyperactivity disorder: A clinical workbook.* New York: Guilford Press.

Barkley, R. A. (1994). Can neuropsychological tests help diagnose ADD/ADHD? *ADHD Report, 1,* 1–3.

Barkley, R. A. (1997). *ADHD and the nature of self-control.* New York: Guilford Press.

Barkley, R. A., & Biederman, J. (1997). Toward a broader definition of the age-of-onset criterion for attention-deficit hyperactivity disorder. *Journal of the American Academy of Child and Adolescent Psychiatry, 36,* 1204–1210.

Barkley, R. A., & Anastopoulos, A. (1992). Adolescents with attention deficit hyperactivity disorder: Mother–adolescent interactions, family beliefs and conflicts, and maternal psychopathology. *Journal of Abnormal Child Psychology, 20,* 263–288.

Barkley, R. A., Fischer, M., Edelbrock, C., & Smallish, L. (1990). The adolescent outcome of hyperactive children diagnosed by research criterion: 1. An 8-year prospective follow-up study. *Journal of the American Academy of Child and Adolescent Psychiatry, 29,* 546–557.

Barkley, R. A., Grodzinsky, G., & DuPaul, G. (1992). Frontal lobe functions in attention deficit disorder with and without hyperactivity: A review and research report. *Journal of Abnormal Child Psychology, 20,* 163–188.

Barkley, R. A., & Murphy, K. (1993). Differential diagnosis of adult ADHD: Some controversial issues. *ADHD Report, 1,* 1–3.

Baumgaertel, A., Wolraich, M., & Dietrich, M. (1995). Comparison of diagnostic criteria for attention deficit disorders in a German elementary school sample. *Journal of the American Academy of Child and Adolescent Psychiatry, 34,* 629–638.

Behar, D. (1984). Sugar challenge testing with children considered behaviorally "sugar reactive." *Nutrition and Behavior, 1,* 277–288.

Bell, N., & Vogel, E. (Eds). (1961). *A modern introduction to the family* (rev. ed.). Glencoe, IL: Free Press.

Bemporad, J., & Zambenedetti, M. (1996). Psychotherapy of adults with attention-deficit disorder. *Journal of Psychotherapy Practice and Research, 5,* 228–237.

Bernard, J. A. (1995). *ADHD and the "freedom of distractibility" factor: Is there a relationship?* Paper presented at the seventh annual meeting of CHADD, Washington, DC.

Berry, R., Shaywitz, E., & Shaywitz, B. (1985). Girls with attention deficit disorder—A silent minority: A report on behavioral and cognitive characteristics. *Pediatrics, 76,* 801–809.

Biederman, J. A., Baldessarini, R., Wright, V., Knee, D., & Harmatz, J. (1989). A double-blind placebo controlled study of desipramine and the treatment of ADD: 1. Efficacy. *Journal of the American Academy of Child and Adolescent Psychiatry, 28,* 777–784.

Biederman, J. A., Faraone, S., Keenan, K., Knee, D., & Tsuang, M. (1990). Family-genetic and psychosocial risk factors in DSM-III attention deficit disorder. *Journal of the American Academy of Child and Adolescent Psychiatry, 29,* 526–533.

Biederman, J. A., Faraone, S., & Lapey, K. (1992). Cormorbidity of diagnosis in attention-deficit hyperactivity disorder. In G. Weiss (Ed.), *Child and adolescent psychiatry clinics of North America: Attention deficit hyperactivity disorder* (pp. 335–360). Philadelphia: Saunders.

Biederman, J. A., Faraone, S., Spencer, T., Wilens, T., Norman, D., & Lapey, K. (1993). Patterns of psychiatric comorbidity, cognition, and psychosocial functioning in adults with attention deficit hyperactivity disorder. *American Journal of Psychiatry, 150,* 1792–1798.

Biederman, J. A., Milberger, S., Faraone, S., Kiely, K., Guite, J., Mick, E., Ablon, S., Warburton, R., & Reed, E. (1995a). Family–environment risk factors for attention-deficit hyperactivity disorder: A test of Rutter's indicators of adversity. *Archives of General Psychiatry, 52,* 464–470.

Biederman, J. A., Munir, K., & Knee, D. (1987). Conduct and oppositional disorder in clinically referred children with attention deficit disorder: A controlled family study. *Journal of the American Academy of Child and Adolescent Psychiatry, 26,* 724–727.

Biederman, J. A., Munir, K., Knee, D., & Habelow, W. (1986). A family study of patients with attention deficit disorder and normal controls. *Journal of Psychiatric Research, 20,* 263–274.

Biederman, J. A., Newcorn, J., & Sprich, S. (1991). Cormorbidity of attention deficit hyperactivity disorder. *American Journal of Psychiatry, 148,* 564–577.

Biederman, J. A., & Steingard, R. (1989). Attention-deficit hyperactivity disorder in adolescents. *Psychiatric Annals, 19,* 587–596.

Biederman, J. A., Wilens, T., Mick, E., & Milberger, S. (1995b). Psychoactive substance use disorders in adults with attention deficit hyperactivity disorder: Effects of ADHD and psychiatric comorbidity. *American Journal of Psychiatry, 152,* 1652–1658.

Borden, K., Brown, R. T., Wynne, M. E., & Schleser, R. (1987). Piagetian conservation and response to cognitive therapy in attention deficit disordered children. *Journal of Child Psychology and Psychiatry and Allied Disciplines, 28,* 755–764.

Boszormenyi-Nagy, I., & Spark, G. (1973). *Invisible loyalties: Reciprocity in intergenerational family therapy.* New York: Harper & Row. (2nd ed. 1984. New York: Brunner/Mazel)

Bowen, M. (1978). *Family therapy in clinical practice.* New York: Aronson.

Brown, R. T., Abramowitz, A., Madan-Swain, A., Eckstrand, D., & Dulcan, M. (1989, August). *ADHD gender differences in a clinical referred sample.* Paper presented at the annual conference of the American Academy of Child and Adolescent Psychiatry, New York, NY.

Brown, R. T., Borden, K., Wynne, M., & Schleser, R. (1986). Methylphenidate and cognitive therapy with ADD children: A methodological reconsideration. *Journal of Abnormal Child Psychology, 14,* 481–497.

Brown, R. T., Borden, K., Wynne, M., & Spunt, A. (1988). Patterns of compliance in a treatment program for children with attention deficit disorder. *Journal of Compliance in Health Care, 3,* 23–39.

Brown, T. E. (1995, October). *Complicated ADDs: Assessment and treatment of comorbidities.* Paper presented at the seventh annual meeting of CHADD, Washington, DC.

Brown, T. E. (1996). *Brown Attention Deficit Disorder Scales.* San Antonio, TX: Psychological Corporation.

Butler, S. F., Arredondo, D., & McCloskey, V. (1995). Affective comorbidity in children and adolescents with attention deficit hyperactivity disorder. *Annals of Clinical Psychiatry, 7,* 51–55.

Cantwell, D. (1972). Psychiatric illness in families of hyperactive children. *Archives of General Psychiatry, 27,* 414–417.

Cantwell, D. (1985). Hyperactive children have grown up: What have we learned about what happens to them? *Archives of General Psychiatry, 42,* 1026–1028.

Cantwell, D. (1988). Families with attention deficit disordered children and others at risk. *Journal of Chemical Dependency Treatment, 1,* 163–186.

Cantwell, D. (1994). *Therapeutic management of attention deficit disorder: Participant workbook.* New York: SCP Communication.

Cantwell, D. (1996). Attention deficit disorder: A review of the past 10 years. *Journal of the American Academy of Child and Adolescent Psychiatry, 35,* 978–987.

Cantwell, D., & Baker, L. (1989). Stability and natural history of DSM-III childhood diagnoses. *Journal of the American Academy of Child and Adolescent Psychiatry, 28,* 691–700.

Carlson, C. L., Lahey, B., & Neeper, R. (1986). Direct assessment of the cognitive correlates of attention deficit disorders with and without hyperactivity. *Journal of Psychopathology and Behavioral Assessment, 8,* 69–86.

Carlson, P. L., Manowitz, P., McBride, H., & Nora, R. (1987). Attention deficit disorder and pathological gambling. *Journal of Clinical Psychiatry, 48*, 487–488.

Castellanos, F., Giedd, J., Marsh, W., Marsh, W., Hamburger, S., Baituzis, A., Dickstein, D., Sarfatti, S., Vauss, Y., Snell, J., Lange, N., Kaysen, D., Drain, A., Ritchie, G., Rajapakse, J., & Rapoport, J. (1996). Quantitative brain magnetic resonance imaging in attention-deficit hyperactivity disorder. *Archives of General Psychiatry, 53*, 607–616.

Chelune, G., Ferguson, W., Koon, R., & Dickey, T. (1986). Frontal lobe disinhibition in attention deficit disorder. *Child Psychiatry and Human Development, 16*, 221–234.

Claude, D., & Firestone, P. (1995). The development of ADHD boys: A 12-year follow-up. *Canadian Journal of Behavioural Sciences, 27*, 226–249.

Cocciarella, A., Wood, R., & Low, K. (1995). Brief behavioral treatment for attention-deficit hyperactivity disorder. *Perceptual and Motor Skills, 8*, 225–226.

Comings, E., Comings, B., & Muhleman, M. (1991). The dopamine D-2 receptor locus as a modifying gene in neuro-psychiatric disorders. *Journal of the American Medical Association, 266*, 1793–1800.

Conners, C. K. (1995). *Conners Adult ADHD History Form.* North Tonawanda, NY: Multi-Health Systems.

Conners, C. K. (1989). *Conners Parent and Teacher Questionnaires.* North Tonawanda, NY: Multi-Health Systems.

Cook, J. R., Mausback, T., Burd, L., & Gascon, G. (1993). A preliminary study of the relationship between central auditory processing disorder and attention deficit disorder. *Journal of Psychiatry and Neuroscience, 18*, 130–137.

Copeland, E. D. (1994). *Copeland Symptom Checklist for Adult Attention Deficit Disorder.* Macon, GA: MCCG Institute for Developmental Medicine.

Costantino, G., Colon-Malgady, G., Malgady, R., & Perez, A. (1991). Assessment of attention deficit disorder using a thematic apperception technique. *Journal of Personality Assessment, 57*, 87–95.

Cousins, L., & Weiss, G. (1993). Parent training and social skills training for children with attention-deficit hyperactivity disorder: How can they be combined for greater effectiveness? *Canadian Journal of Psychiatry, 38*, 449–457.

Culbert, T., Banex, G., & Reiff, M. (1994). Children who have attentional disorders: Interventions. *Pediatrics in Review, 15*, 5–15.

Culbertson, J., & Silovsky, J. (1996). Learning disabilities and attention deficit hyperactivity disorder: Their impact on children's significant others. In F. Kaslow (Ed.), *Handbook of relational diagnosis and dysfunctional family patterns* (pp. 186–210). New York: Wiley.

Davila, R., Williams, M., & MacDonald, J. (1991). *Clarification of policy to address the needs of children with attention deficit disorders within general and/or special education.* Washington, DC: U.S. Department of Education.

Dicks, H. (1967). *Marital tension.* New York: Basic Books.

Dixon, E. B. (1995). Impact of adult ADD on the family. In K. G. Nadeau (Ed.), *A comprehensive guide to attention deficit disorder in adults: Research, diagnosis, and treatment* (pp. 236–259). New York: Brunner/Mazel.

Douglas, V. (1984). The psychological processes implicated in ADD. In L. M.

Bloomingdale (Ed.), *Attention deficit disorder: Diagnostic, cognitive, and therapeutic understanding* (pp. 78–96). New York: Spectrum.

Edwards, M., Schulz, E., & Long, N. (1995). The role of the family in the assessment of attention deficit hyperactivity disorder. *Clinical Psychology Review, 15,* 375–394.

Erhardt, D., & Baker, B. (1990). The effects of behavioral parent training on families with young hyperactive children. *Journal of Behavioral Therapy and Experimental Psychiatry, 21,* 121–132.

Estrada, A., & Pinsoff, W. (1995). The effectiveness of family therapies for selected behavioral disorders of childhood. *Journal of Marital and Family Therapy, 21,* 403–440.

Everett, C. A., Halperin, S., Volgy, S., & Wissler, A. (1989). *Treating the borderline family: A systemic approach.* New York: Allyn & Bacon.

Everett, C. A., & Volgy, S. (1983). Family assessment in child custody disputes. *Journal of Marital and Family Therapy, 9,* 342–355.

Everett, C. A., & Volgy-Everett, S. (1998). *Short-term therapy with borderline patients and their families.* Iowa City, IA: Geist & Russell.

Eyre, S., Rounsaville, B., & Kleber, H. (1982). History of childhood hyperactivity in a clinical population of opiate addicts. *Journal of Nervous and Mental Disorders, 170,* 522–529.

Faigel, H., Sznajderman, S., Tishby, O., & Turel, M. (1995). Attention deficit disorder during adolescence: A review. *Journal of Adolescent Health, 16,* 174–184.

Faraone, S., Biederman, J., Keenan, K., & Ysuang, M. (1991). A family–genetic study of girls with DSM-III attention deficit disorder. *American Journal of Psychiatry, 148,* 112–117.

Faraone, S., Biederman, J., & Milberger, S. (1995). How reliable are maternal reports of their children's psychopathology? One-year recall of psychiatric diagnoses of ADHD children. *Journal of the American Academy of Child and Adolescent Psychiatry, 34,* 1001–1008.

Fehlings, D. L., Roberts, W., Humphries, T., & Dawe, G. (1991). Attention deficit hyperactivity disorder: Does cognitive behavioral therapy improve home behavior? *Journal of Developmental and Behavioral Pediatrics, 12,* 223–228.

Framo, J. L. (1992). *Family-of-origin-therapy: An intergenerational approach.* New York: Brunner/Mazel.

Frick, P. J., Lahey, B., Christ, M., & Loeber, R. (1991). History of childhood behavior problems in biological relatives of boys with attention-deficit hyperactivity disorder and conduct disorder. *Journal of Clinical Child Psychology, 20,* 445–451.

Gabel, S., Schmitz, S., & Fulker, D. (1996). Comorbidity in hyperactive children: Issues related to selection bias, gender, severity, and internalizing symptoms. *Child Psychiatry and Human Development, 27,* 15–28.

Gadow, K., & Sprafkin, J. (1994). *Child Symptom Inventories.* Stony Brook, NY: Checkmate Plus.

Gadow, K., & Sprafkin, J. (1996, April). *Assessing comorbidities in children with ADHD.* Paper presented at the annual meeting of the National Association of School Psychologists, Atlanta, GA.

Gascon, G. G., Johnson, R., & Burd, L. (1986). Central auditory processing and attention deficit disorders. *Journal of Child Neurology, 1,* 27–33.

Gilles, J., Gilger, J., Pennington, B., & DeFries, J. (1992). Attention deficit disorder in reading-disabled twins: Evidence for a genetic etiology. *Journal of Abnormal Child Psychology, 20,* 303–315.

Gittelman, R., Mannuzza, S., Shenker, R., & Bonagura, N. (1985). Hyperactive boys almost grown-up: 1. Psychiatric status. *Archives of General Psychiatry, 42,* 937–947.

Goodman, R., & Stevenson, J. (1989). A twin study of hyperactivity: 2. The aetiological role of genes, family relationships, and perinatal adversity. *Journal of Child Psychology and Psychiatry, 30,* 691–709.

Gordon, M. (1986). How is a computerized attention test used in the diagnosis of attention deficit disorder? *Journal of Children in a Contemporary Society, 19,* 53–64.

Gordon, M., & Metelman, B. (1988). The assessment of attention: 1. Standardization and reliability of a behavior-based measure. *Journal of Clinical Psychology, 44,* 682–690.

Greenberg, L., & Waldman, I. (1993). Developmental normative data on the test of variables of attention (T.O.V.A.). *Journal of Child Psychology and Psychiatry and Allied Disciplines, 34,* 1019–1030.

Halikas, J., Meller, J., Morce, C., & Lyttle, M. (1990). Predicting substance abuse in juvenile offenders: Attention deficit disorder versus aggressivity. *Child Psychology and Human Development, 21,* 49–55.

Hallowell, E. M., & Ratey, J. J. (1994). *Driven to distraction.* New York: Pantheon Books.

Halperin, J., Wolf, L., Pascualvaca, D., & Newcorn, J. (1988). Differential assessment of attention and impulsivity in children. *Journal of the American Academy of Child and Adolescent Psychiatry, 27,* 326–329.

Hartmann, T. (1993). *Attention deficit disorder: A different perception.* Novato, CA: Underwood-Miller Press.

Hartsough, C., & Lambert, N. (1982). Some environmental and familial correlates and antecedents of hyperactivity. *American Journal of Orthopsychiatry, 52,* 272–287.

Harvey, J. R., & Chernouskas, C. (1995, October). *Diagnosis and description of attention deficit/hyperactivity disorder with the Woodcock Johnson Psychoeducational Battery-Revised.* Paper presented at the seventh annual meeting of CHADD, Washington, DC.

Heath, C., & Kush, J. (1991). Use of discrepancy formulas in the assessment of learning disability. In J. E. Obrzut & G. W. Hund (Eds.), *Neuropsychological foundations of learning disabilities* (pp. 287–307). San Diego: Academic Press.

Hechtman, L. (1996). Families of children with attention deficit hyperactivity disorder: A review. *Canadian Journal of Psychiatry, 41,* 350–360.

Henry, G. (1987). Symbolic modeling and parent behavioral training: Effects on noncompliance of hyperactive children. *Journal of Behavior Therapy and Experimental Psychiatry, 18,* 105–113.

Hinshaw, S., Buhrmester, D., & Heller, T. (1989). Anger control in response to verbal provocation: Effects of stimulant medication for boys with ADHD. *Journal of Abnormal Child Psychology, 17,* 393–407.

Holdnack, J. A., Moberg, P., Arnold, S., & Gur, R. (1994). MMPI characteristics in adults diagnosed with ADD: A preliminary report. *International Journal of Neuroscience, 79,* 47–58.

Holdnack, J. A., Moberg, P., Arnold, S., Gur, R., & Gur, R. (1995). Speed of processing and verbal learning deficits in adults diagnosed with attention deficit disorder. *Neuropsychiatry, Neuropsychology and Behavioral Neurology, 8,* 282–292.

Hopkins, J., Perlman, T., Hechtman, L., & Weiss, G. (1979). Cognitive styles in adults originally diagnosed as hyperactives. *Journal of Child Psychology and Psychiatry, 20,* 209–216.

Hoza, B., & Pelham, W. (1995). Social–cognitive predictors of treatment response in children with ADHD. *Journal of Social and Clinical Psychology, 14,* 23–35.

Huessy, H., & Howell, D. (1985). Relationship between adult alcoholism and childhood behavior disorders. *Psychiatric Journal of the University of Ottawa, 10,* 114–119.

Hussey, H. R. (1990). *The pharmacotherapy of personality disorder in women.* A paper presented to the annual meeting of the American Psychiatric Association, New York, NY.

Hynd, G., Semund-Clikeman, M., Lorys, A., Novey, E., & Eliopulos, D. (1990). Brain morphology in development dyslexia and attention deficit disorder hyperactivity. *Archives of Neurology, 47,* 919–926.

Interagency Committee on Learning Disabilities. (1987). *Learning disabilities: A report to the U. S. Congress.* Washington, DC: U. S. Government Printing Office.

Jaffe, S. L. (1991). Intranasal abuse of prescribed methylphenidate by an alcohol and drug abusing adolescent with ADHD. *Journal of the American Academy of Child and Adolescent Psychiatry, 30,* 505–523.

Jensen, J., Burke, N., & Garfinkel, B. (1988). Depression and symptoms of attention deficit disorder with hyperactivity. *Journal of the American Academy of Child and Adolescent Psychiatry, 27,* 742–747.

Jerome, L. (1995). "Comorbidity of central auditory processing disorder and attention-deficit hyperactivity disorder": Comment. *Journal of the American Academy of Child and Adolescent Psychiatry, 34,* 126–127.

Johnson, C. (1996). Parent characteristics and parent–child interactions in families of nonproblem children and ADHD children with higher and lower levels of oppositional-defiant behavior. *Journal of Abnormal Child Psychology, 24,* 85–104.

Johnson, C., & Behrenz, K. (1993). Childrearing discussions in families of nonproblem children and ADHD children with higher and lower levels of aggressive-defiant behaviors. *Canadian Journal of School Psychology, 9,* 53–65.

Kaufman, A. (1980). Issues in psychological assessment: Interpreting the WISC-R intelligently. In B. Lahey & A. Kazdin (Eds.), *Advances in clinical child psychology* (Vol. 3, pp. 177–214). New York: Plenum Press.

Kelly, K. (1995). Adult ADD support groups. In K. G. Nadeau (Ed.), *A comprehen-*

sive guide to attention deficit disorder in adults: Research, diagnosis, and treatment (pp. 352–374). New York: Brunner/Mazel.

Klee, S. H. (1986). The clinical psychological evaluation of attention deficit disorder. *Psychiatric Annals, 16,* 43–46.

Klorman, R., Brumaghim, J., Fitzpatrick, P., & Borgstedt, A. (1991). Methylphenidate speeds evaluation processes of attention deficit disorder adolescents during continuous performance test. *Journal of Abnormal Child Psychology, 19,* 263–283.

Kramer, J. (1986). What are hyperactive children like as young adults? *Journal of Children in a Contemporary Society, 19,* 89–98.

Kuehne, C., Kehle, T., & McMahon, W. (1987). Differences between children with attention deficit disorder, children with specific learning disabilities, and normal children. *Journal of School Psychology, 25,* 161–166.

Lahey, B., Schaughency, E., Hynd, G., Carlson, C., & Nieves, N. (1987). Attention deficit disorder with and without hyperactivity: Comparison of behavioral characteristics of clinic-referred children. *Journal of the Academy of Child and Adolescent Psychiatry, 26,* 718–723.

Latham, P. S., & Latham, P. H. (1995). Legal rights of the ADD adult. In K. G. Nadeau (Ed.), *A comprehensive guide to attention deficit disorder in adults: Research, diagnosis, and treatment* (pp. 337–351). New York: Brunner/Mazel.

Levine, M. (1985). *The ANSER system.* Cambridge, MA: Educators Publishing Service.

Linden, M., Habib, T., & Radojevic, V. (1996). A controlled study of the effects of EEG biofeedback on cognition and behavior of children with attention deficit disorder and learning disabilities. *Biofeedback and Self-Regulation, 21,* 35–49.

Loeber, R., Green, S., & Keenan, K. (1995). Which boys will fare worse? Early predictors of the onset of conduct disorder and hyperactivity. *Journal of the American Academy of Child and Adolescent Psychiatry, 34,* 499–509.

Lomas, B. (1995). Diagnosing attention deficit hyperactivity disorder in adults. *American Journal of Psychiatry, 152,* 961–962.

Lubar, J., Bianchine, K., Calhoun, H., Lambert, E., Brody, Z., & Nielsen, J. (1985). Special analysis of EEG differences between children with and without learning disabilities. *Journal of Learning Disabilities, 18,* 403–408.

Mannuzza, S., Klein, R., Bonagura, N., Malloy, P., Giampino, T., & Addalli, K. (1991). Hyperactive boys almost grown up: V. Replication of psychiatric status. *Archives of General Psychiatry, 48,* 77–83.

Mannuzza, S., Klein, R., Bessler, A., Malloy, P., & Hynes, M. (1997). Educational and occupational outcome of hyperactive boys grown up. *Journal of the American Academy of Child and Adolescent Psychiatry, 36,* 1222–1227.

Mannuzza, S., Klien, R., Bessler, A., Malloy, P., & LaPadula, M. (1993). Adult outcome of hyperactive boys: Educational achievement, occupational rank, and psychiatric status. *Archives of General Psychiatry, 50,* 575–576.

Marshall, V., Longwell, L., Goldstein, M., & Swanson, J. (1990). Family factors associated with aggressive symptomatology in boys with attention deficit hyperactivity disorder: A research note. *Journal of Child Psychology and Psychiatry, 31,* 629–636.

McBurnett, K. (1995). The new subtype of ADHD: Predominantly hyperactive-impulsive. *Attention, 1,* 10–15.

McCarney, S. (1995). *Attention Deficit Disorders Evaluation Scale.* Columbia, MO: Hawthorne Educational Services.

McGee, R., Stanton, W., & Sears, M. (1993). Allergic disorders and attention deficit disorder in children. *Journal of Abnormal Child Psychology, 21,* 79–88.

McGee, R., Williams, S., & Feehan, M. (1992). Attention deficit disorder and age of onset of problem behaviors. *Journal of Abnormal Child Psychology, 20,* 487–502.

Miller, K. J. (1994, October). *Medication for attention deficit disorder: A guide for parent and educators.* Paper presented at the sixth annual meeting of CHADD, New York, NY.

Minuchin, S. (1974). *Families and family therapy.* Cambridge, MA: Harvard University Press.

Minuchin, S., & Fishman, H. (1981). *Family therapy techniques.* Cambridge, MA: Harvard University Press.

Moffitt, T., & Silva, P. (1988). Self-reported delinquency, neuropsychological deficit, and history of attention deficit disorder. *Journal of Abnormal Child Psychology, 16,* 553–569.

Molt, L. F. (1996). An examination of various aspects of auditory processing in clutterers. *Journal of Fluency Disorders, 21,* 215–225.

Morgan, A., Hynd, G., Riccio, C., & Hall, J. (1996). Validity of DSM-IV ADHD predominantly inattentive and combined types: Relationship to previous DSM diagnoses/subtype differences. *Journal of the American Academy of Child and Adolescent Psychiatry, 35,* 325–333.

Morrison, J., & Stewart, M. (1971). Family study of the hyperactive child syndrome. *Biological Psychiatry, 3,* 189–195.

Morrison, J., & Stewart, M. (1973). Evidence of polygenic inheritance in the hyperactive child syndrome. *American Journal of Psychiatry, 130,* 791–792.

Munir, K., Biederman, J., & Knee, D. (1987). Psychiatric comorbidity in patients with attention deficit disorder: A controlled study. *Journal of the American Academy of Child and Adolescent Psychiatry, 26,* 844–848.

Murphy, K. R. (1995). *Out of the fog: Treatment options and coping strategies for adult attention-deficit disorder.* New York: Hyperion.

Nadeau, K. G. (1995a). ADD in the workplace: Career consultation and counseling. In K. G. Nadeau (Ed.), *A comprehensive guide to attention deficit disorder in adults: Research, diagnosis, and treatment* (pp. 308–334). New York: Brunner/Mazel.

Nadeau, K. G. (1995b). *Adult ADHD Questionnaire.* Annandale, VA: Chesapeake Psychological Publishers.

Nadeau, K. G. (1997). *ADD in the workplace: Choices, changes, and challenges.* New York: Brunner/Mazel.

Nichols, W. C., & Everett, C. A. (1987). *Systemic family therapy: An integrative approach.* New York: Guilford Press.

O'Brien, J., Halperin, J., Newcorn, J., Sharma, V., et al. (1992). Psychometric differentiation of conduct disorder and attention deficit disorder with hyperactivity. *Journal of Developmental and Behavioral Pediatrics, 13,* 274–277.

O'Brien, J., Phillips, W., & Stein, M. (1994). *Gender differences in attention deficit hyperactivity disorder and attention deficit disorder-undifferentiated.* Paper presented at the fifth annual meeting of CHADD, San Diego, CA.

Pantle, M., Ebner, D., & Hynan, L. (1994). The Rorschach and the assessment of impulsivity. *Journal of Clinical Psychology, 50,* 633–638.

Paternite, C., Loney, J., & Roberts, M. A. (1995). External validation of oppositional disorder and attention deficit disorder with hyperactivity. *Journal of Abnormal Child Psychology, 23,* 453–471.

Payne, N. (1994, October). *Romancing the inattentive: Assessing the ADHD symptomatic behaviors in the intimate relationships of diagnosed adults.* Poster presented at the fifth annual meeting of CHADD, New York, NY.

Pelham, W., Swanson, J., Furman, M., & Schwindt, H. (1995). Pemoline effect on children with ADHD: A time-response by dose–response analysis on classroom measures. *Journal of the American Academy of Child and Adolescent Psychiatry, 34,* 1504–1513.

Phillips, W., Gutermuth, L., O'Brien, J., Szumowski, B., & Stein, M. (1993). *Gender differences in attention deficit hyperactivity disorder: Cognitive and behavioral characteristics.* Paper presented at the annual meeting of the American Psychological Society, Chicago, IL.

Pisterman, S., Firestone, P., McGrath, P., Goodman, J., Webster, I., Mallory, R., & Goffin, B. (1992). The role of parent training in treatment of preschoolers with ADDH. *American Journal of Orthopsychiatry, 62,* 397–408.

Pisterman, S., McGrath, P., Firestone, P., & Goodman, J. (1989). Outcome of parent-mediated treatment of preschoolers with attention deficit disorder with hyperactivity. *Journal of Consulting and Clinical Psychology, 57,* 636–643.

Popper, C. W. (1989). Diagnosing bipolar vs. ADHD. *Newsletter of the American Academy of Child and Adolescent Psychiatry, Summer,* 5–6.

Prescott, D. (1993). The relative validity of a computer attention test and teacher rating scales to predict attention deficit disorder and other diagnostic categories. *Dissertation Abstracts International, 53,* 3789.

Quinn, P. (1997). *Attention deficit disorder: Diagnosis and treatment from infancy to adulthood.* New York: Brunner/Mazel.

Reiff, M., Banez, G., & Culbert, T. (1993). Children who have attentional disorders: Diagnosis and evaluation. *Pediatric Review, 12,* 455–465.

Robin, A. L. (1998). *ADHD in adolescents: Diagnosis and treatment.* New York: Guilford Press.

Robin, A. L., Bedway, M., Tzelepis, A., & Gilroy, M. (1995, October). *Impact of multiple ADHD on the family: A descriptive study.* Poster presented at the seventh annual meeting of CHADD, Washington, DC.

Roth, N., Beyreiss, J., Schlenzka, K., & Beyer, H. (1991). Coincidence of attention deficit disorder and atopic disorders in children: Empirical findings and hypothetical background. *Journal of Abnormal Child Psychology, 19,* 1–13.

Routh, D. K. (1983). Attention deficit disorder: Its relationship with activity, aggression, and achievement. *Advances in Developmental and Behavioral Pediatrics, 4,* 125–163.

Satterfield, J., Swanson, J., Schell, A., & Lee, F. (1994). Prediction of antisocial behavior in attention-deficit hyperactivity disorder boys from aggression/defiant scores. *Journal of the American Academy of Child and Adolescent Psychiatry, 33,* 185–190.

Sattler, J. (1988). *Assessment of children* (3rd ed.). San Diego: J. M. Sattler.

Schubiner, H., & Tzelepis, A. (1996, May). *Treating the substance abusing adult with ADD.* Paper presented at the second annual meeting if the National Attention Deficit Disorder Association Adult ADD Conference, Pittsburgh, PA.

Schubiner, H., Tzelepis, A., Isaacson, J., Warbasse, L., Zachorek, M., & Musial, J. (1995). The dual diagnosis of attention-deficit/hyperactivity disorder and substance abuse: Case reports and literature review. *Journal of Clinical Psychiatry, 56,* 146–150.

Seidel, W., & Joschko, M. (1990). Evidence of difficulties in sustained attention in children with ADDH. *Journal of Abnormal Child Psychology, 18,* 217–229.

Seidel, W., & Joschko, M. (1991). Assessment of attention in children. *Clinical Neuropsychologist, 5,* 53–66.

Seidman, L., Biederman, J., Faraone, S., Milberger, S., Norman, D., Ceiberd, K., Benedict, K., Guite, J., Mick, E., & Kiely, K. (1995). Effects of family history and comorbidity on the neuropsychological performance of children with ADHD: Preliminary findings. *Journal of the American Academy of Child and Adolescent Psychiatry, 34,* 1015–1024.

Shaywitz, S., & Shaywitz, B. (1988). Attention deficit disorder: Current perspectives. In J. Kavanaugh & T. Truss (Eds.), *Learning disabilities: Proceedings* (pp. 369–523). Parkton, MD: York Press.

Shekim, W., Asarnow, R., Hess, E., Aaucha, K., & Wheeler, N. (1990). A clinical and demographic profile of a sample of adults with attention deficit hyperactivity disorder, residual state. *Comprehensive Psychiatry, 31,* 416–425.

Simeon, J., Ferguson, H., & Van Wyck Fleet, J. (1986). Bupropion effects in attention deficit and conduct disorders. *Canadian Journal of Psychiatry, 31,* 581–585.

Soltys, S., Kashani, J., Dandoy, A., & Vaidya, A. (1992). Comorbidity for disruptive behavior disorders in psychiatrically hospitalized children. *Child Psychiatry and Human Development, 23,* 87–98.

Spencer, T., Biederman, J., Wilens, T., Faraone, S., & Li, T. (1994). Is attention deficit hyperactivity disorder in adults a valid diagnosis? *Harvard Review of Psychiatry, 1,* 326–335.

Stierlin, H. (1973). A family perspective on adolescent runaways. *Archives of General Psychiatry, 12,* 56–62.

Stierlin, H. (1974). *Separating parents and adolescents: A perspective on running away, schizophrenia, and waywardness.* New York: Quadrangle.

Strober, M. (1996). Childhood onset of bipolar disorder: Identification and treatment. *Psychiatric Times Bipolar Disorders Letter, 2,* 1–3.

Summers, J., & Caplan, P. (1987). Laypeople's attitudes toward drug treatment for behavioral control depend on which disorder and which drug. *Clinical Pediatrics, 26,* 258–262.

Triolo, S. J. (1995). *Attention-Deficit Scales for Adults.* New York: Brunner/Mazel.

Tzelepis, A. (1997, February). *Diagnosing ADHD in adults.* Paper presented to the third annual meeting of the National Attention Deficit Disorder Association, St. Louis, MO.

Tzelepis, A., & Schubiner, H. (1995, October). *Psychiatric comorbidity and psychosocial functioning in adults with attention deficit hyperactivity disorder.* Paper presented at the sixth annual meeting of CHADD, New York, NY.

Tzelepis, A., Schubiner, H., & Warbasse, L. (1994). Differential diagnosis and psychiatric co-morbidity patterns in adult attention deficit disorder. In K. G. Nadeau (Ed.), *A comprehensive guide to attention deficit disorders in adults* (pp. 280–309). New York: Brunner/Mazel.

Ullmann, R. K. (1985). ACTeRS useful in screening learning disabled from attention deficit disordered (ADD-H) children. *Psychopharmacology Bulletin, 21,* 547–551.

Ullmann, R. K., Sleator, E., & Sprague, R. (1984). A new rating scale for diagnosis and monitoring of ADD children. *Psychopharmacology Bulletin, 20,* 160–164.

Ullmann, R. K., Sleator, E., & Sprague, R. (1990). *ADD Comprehensive Teacher Rating Scale.* Champaign, IL: Metritech.

Vandermay, S., & Robin, A. L. (1994). *Adolescent self-report of ADHD symptoms.* Poster presented at the fifth annual meeting of CHADD, New York, NY.

van der Vlugt, H., Pijnenburg, H., Wels, P., & Koning, A. (1995). Cognitive behavior modification of ADHD: A family system approach. In H. van Bilsen, P. Kendall, & J. Slavenburg (Eds.), *Behavioral approaches for children and adolescents: Challenges for the next century* (pp. 65–75). New York: Plenum Press.

Walker, J., Lahey, B., Hynd, G., & Frame, C. (1987). Comparison of specific patterns of antisocial behavior in children with conduct disorder with or without coexisting hyperactivity. *Journal of Consulting and Clinical Psychology, 55,* 910–913.

Warneke, L. (1990). Psychostimulants in psychiatry. *Canadian Journal of Psychiatry, 35,* 3–10.

Weiss, G., Hechtman, L., Milroy, T., & Perlman, T. (1985). Psychiatric status of hyperactives as adults: A controlled prospective 15-year follow-up of 63 hyperactive children. *Journal of the American Academy of Child Psychiatry, 23,* 211–220.

Weiss, L. (1994). *The attention deficit disorder in adults workbook.* Dallas, TX: Taylor.

Wender, E. (1985). The Utah criteria in diagnosing attention deficit disorder. *Psychopharmacology Bulletin, 21,* 222–231.

Wender, E. (1995). Attention-deficit hyperactivity disorders in adolescence. *Journal of Developmental and Behavioral Pediatrics, 16,* 192–195.

Wender, P. H. (1995). *Attention-deficit hyperactivity disorder in adults.* New York: Oxford University Press.

Wender, P. H., Reimherr, F., Wood, D., & Ward, M. (1985). A controlled study of methylphenidate in the treatment of attention deficit disorder, residual type, in adults. *American Journal of Psychiatry, 142,* 547–552.

Wender, P. H., & Reimherr, F. (1990). Bupropion treatment of attention deficit hyperactivity disorder in adults. *American Journal of Psychiatry, 147,* 1018–1020.

Wilens, T. E. (1998). *Straight talk about psychiatric medications for kids*. New York: Guilford Press.

Wilens, T. E., & Biederman, J. (1992). The stimulants. In D. Shafer (Ed.), *The psychiatric clinics of North America* (pp. 191–222). Philadelphia: Saunders.

Wilens, T. E., Biederman, J., Spencer, T., & Frances, R. (1994). Comorbidity of attention deficit hyperactivity disorder and the psychoactive substance use disorders. *Hospital and Community Psychiatry, 45,* 421–435.

Wilens, T. E., Biederman, J., Spencer, T., & Prince, J. (1995a). Pharmacotherapy of adult attention deficit/hyperactivity disorder: A review. *Journal of Clinical Psychopharmacology, 15,* 270–279.

Wilens, T. E., & Lineham, C. (1995). ADD and substance abuse: An intoxicating combination. *Attention, 3,* 24–31.

Wilens, T. E., Prince, J., Biederman, J., & Spencer, T. (1995b). Attention-deficit hyperactivity disorder and comorbid substance use disorders in adults. *Psychiatric Services, 46,* 761–763.

Wolraich, M., Hannah, J., Pinnock, T., Baumgartel, A., & Brown, J. (1996). Comparison of diagnostic criteria for attention-deficit hyperactivity disorder in a county-wide sample. *Journal of the American Academy of Child and Adolescent Psychiatry, 35,* 319–324.

Wood, D., Wender, P., & Reimherr, F. (1983). The prevalence of attention deficit disorder, residual type, or minimal brain dysfunction, in a population of male alcoholic patients. *American Journal of Psychiatry, 140,* 95–98.

Zagar, R., Arbit, J., Hughes, J., & Busell, R. (1989). Developmental and disruptive behavior disorders among delinquents. *Journal of the American Academy of Child and Adolescent Psychiatry, 28,* 437–440.

Zametkin, A., Liebenauer, L., Fitzgerald, G., & King, A. (1993). Brain metabolism in teenagers with attention-deficit hyperactivity disorder. *Archives of General Psychiatry, 50,* 333–340.

Zametkin, A., Gross, M., King, A., Semple, W., Rumsey, J., Hamburger, S., & Cohen, R. (1990). Cerebral glucose metabolism in adults with hyperactivity childhood onset. *New England Journal of Medicine, 323,* 1361–1366.

Zametkin, A., & Rapoport, J. (1987). Neurobiology of attention deficit disorder with hyperactivity: Where have we come in 50 years? *Journal of the American Academy of Child and Adolescent Psychiatry, 26,* 676–686.

Zarski, J., Cook, R., West, J., & O'Keefe, S. (1987). Attention deficit disorder: Identification and assessment issues. *American Mental Health Counselors Association Journal, 9,* 3–13.

Index